THE HANDHOLDER'S HANDBOOK

The Handholder's Handbook

A GUIDE
FOR CAREGIVERS OF PEOPLE
WITH ALZHEIMER'S OR OTHER DEMENTIAS

ROSETTE TEITEL

Rutgers University Press
New Brunswick, New Jersey, and London

Library of Congress Cataloging-in-Publication Data

Teitel, Rosette, 1939–
    The handholder's handbook : a guide for caregivers of people with
Alzheimer's or other dementias / Rosette Teitel.
        p.   cm.
    Includes bibliographical references and index.
    ISBN 0-8135-2939-5 (cloth) — ISBN 0-8135-2940-9 (pbk.)
    1. Alzheimer's disease—Patients—Care—Handbooks, manuals, etc.
2. Alzheimer's disease—Patients—Family relationships—Handbooks,
manuals, etc.   3. Caregivers—Handbooks, manuals, etc.   I. Title.
    RC523.2.T45   2001
    362.1'9683—dc21

                                                            00-045680
British Cataloging-in-Publication data for this book is available from the
British Library.

Manufactured in the United States of America

To my beloved husband, Newton,
who taught me so much

CONTENTS

FOREWORD

As a neurologist who has been involved in the care of patients with Alzheimer's disease and other forms of dementia for many years, I pride myself on my expertise and flatter myself to think that my job is a demanding one. It is humbling to be reminded how much more difficult is the task of caring for someone you love with dementia, and how inadequate the professional advice of a physician may be to the caregiver. Alzheimer's disease afflicts the caregiver more in some respects than the patient. The caregivers of patients with Alzheimer's disease are more likely to require medical care or become depressed than other people their age. They shoulder an enormous and unrelenting burden.

While there are many books out there targeted at the millions of people who care for patients with Alzheimer's and other dementing illnesses, this one is unique. Rosette Teitel has written a courageous and informative caregiver's guide from the perspective of someone who has been there and done that. It is like a portable support group. For every issue that threatens to overwhelm you, there is a calm, reassuring, and pragmatic response. Moreover, she anticipates the problems you are likely to encounter, affording you the opportunity to cope with them before they escalate into crises.

The opening chapter provides a clear and concise overview of the diagnosis and available treatment options for Alzheimer's disease. With this background in place, Teitel goes on to describe the effects of the disease on the patient and the caregiver as it progresses. There is a wealth of practical information and advice about physical techniques, support groups, social services, home health aides, nursing homes, insurance, and estate planning. In addition to preparing you to care for the patient, an emphasis is placed on how to take care of yourself. Accordingly, the scope of this book extends beyond caring for the patient at the end of life, through grieving and survival thereafter.

A remarkable attribute of this book is that it manages to be at the same time both intensely personal and generalizable. In order to broaden its perspective, there is a chapter devoted to interviews with adult children of parents with dementia. Other chapters include memorable comments overheard at support group meetings and answers to frequently asked questions. Finally, the resources at the end of the book provide essential charts and forms and an extensive list of agencies and organizations, as well as Internet sites, that may supply further information or assistance.

The Handholder's Handbook is an invaluable resource for the caregiver. It contains the solace and insight to make this difficult process more manageable. We should all be grateful to the author for sharing her hard-won wisdom with us.

Marc L. Gordon, M.D.

Chief of Neurology, Hillside Hospital,
Long Island Jewish Medical Center

Assistant Professor of Neurology
and Psychiatry, Albert Einstein
College of Medicine

PREFACE

My husband, Newton, died of complications from his many ailments, including vascular dementia. It was January 5, the beginning of a new year.

When Newton was admitted to the hospital ten months earlier with acute heart failure, I had no idea that I was in for the toughest learning experience of my life. One of his many health problems was lack of thyroid function, which affected his ability to think clearly.

That symptom didn't show itself at first, but one day, while we were waiting for the thyroid count to go up enough to even do an angiogram, Newton sounded "cuckoo," as I called it. He was, to put it politely, confused. However, he realized it and bounced back to being himself. The next time it happened, he said something the next day about having really been "out of it." So, although it was puzzling, I didn't see it as a cause for alarm. I concentrated on the upcoming open heart surgery. He was considered a high-risk patient, and when he came through without being on a respirator in the recovery room, I was thrilled. His incision healed slowly. Following some complications, he was home after a nine-week absence.

One of the attending physicians in the hospital shocked me by using the term "dementia." I was indignant: I thought, Newton wasn't demented, he was only reacting to powerful medication. (He was, but that wasn't the only problem.) In the long run, the diagnosis of dementia turned out to be right.

Thanks to Medicare, we had wonderful help at home for four hours a day for a few weeks. Newton regained some strength, and he slowly became physically more independent. At the same time, however, he became mentally more confused, even after some of the offending medication was tapered down or eliminated. He'd have good days and bad days, yet he was still functioning. On the day of his seventieth birthday celebration, he was in great form, and the world looked rosy. It was an illusion. His dementia was growing. It eventually took over his entire being. Little by little, he was unable to wash himself, walk unassisted, control his bodily functions, or, at the very end, even feed himself.

His doctors gave me no clue as to what I could expect. Once it became obvious that the damage was irreversible, I didn't realize that meant there would be a downhill slide that would leave poor Newton a shell of himself, and me a physical and emotional wreck. I needed a guide of some kind. Where to turn? How do you give a 170-pound man a shower? How do you deal with his exaggerated fear of falling? How do you pick him up when he does fall? There were so many challenges that crept out of every day. There were so few sources of information.

That is why, now that Newton is gone, I want to give other caregivers the help the members of my support group and I couldn't find. I have tried to make this an easy-to-read guide. Hopefully, this book will answer most questions before they even come up and will enable you to make the decisions that are right for you and your patient. It is aimed at caregivers of those who are already past the beginning stages of the disease.

I have consulted a number of professionals, and their input makes it possible to give you a truly informed and accurate picture of your options. I hope all this can lighten your load just a little.

You are constantly holding the hand of your afflicted loved one. Who is there to hold your hand? I hope this handbook will give you some of the support you need, at any time of the day or night, and hold your hand, in effect.

The checklists at the end of each chapter summarize the discussion and provide reminders for what you need to do next, and the suggested reading lists will enable you to explore a particular topic more thoroughly.

It is my sincere hope that this handbook will give you comfort and perspective. I've been there, and I can assure you that there really is a light at the end of the tunnel. You will come out of this darkness. I send you my caring and support.

Rosette Teitel
Douglaston, New York
August 2000

ACKNOWLEDGMENTS

My gratitude goes first to Justine Ramnarine, without whose help this book would not have seen the light of day. Thanks also to my son, Michael, whose patience and computer knowledge enabled me to start this project and bring the manuscript to completion. My daughter, Ellen, gave me excellent advice all along the way. To all my friends who offered support and encouragement, thank you.

The following caring and knowledgeable professionals contributed their expertise: Dr. Marc L. Gordon, Dr. David Narov, Dr. Greg Hinrichsen, and Steven H. Stern, Esq. Their guidance was invaluable.

Chapter 9 was born because the adult children of a variety of dementia patients were willing to confide their most private thoughts and emotions. I am grateful to them.

I am indebted to Helen Hsu of Rutgers University Press for her faith in the value of this book, and to Suzanne Kellam for her guidance.

Finally, the members of my Alzheimer's support group and our superb leader, Elisabeth Savarese, M.S.W., inspired me to create *The Handholder's Handbook*, while Michele Pinto gave me the information that enabled me to get started.

THE HANDHOLDER'S HANDBOOK

CHAPTER 1

Diagnosis, Progression of the Disease, Treatments, and Alternatives

Things just haven't been quite right for a long time now. You suspected, you really dreaded, that it might be Alzheimer's disease, but you kept putting off a definite diagnosis. Actually, no diagnosis is 100 percent accurate. Until recently, it was arrived at only by a process of elimination, of exclusion. Now it is possible to diagnose Alzheimer's with 85 percent accuracy using methods of inclusion. A pattern that is distinct from other memory distortions can be identified by a trained physician as characteristic of Alzheimer's disease. Alzheimer's is a form of dementia, but not all dementias are Alzheimer's. Dementia is a syndrome, not a disease. That is, it shows itself by a group of symptoms. There are many diseases that can cause the syndrome of dementia.

In my interview with Dr. Marc L. Gordon, chief of neurology of the Hillside Hospital Division of Long Island Jewish Medical Center in New Hyde Park, New York, I learned that dementia can be caused by a stroke, circulatory problems, head trauma, lead poisoning, or medication. Dementia can be attributed to degenerative, vascular, traumatic, or toxic causes. Someone with dementia has problems in more than one area of functioning. These problems represent an acquired loss of skills that the person had previously. The skills are impaired to the point where you know it's more than the normal aging process. This impairment interferes with the ability to function. It takes time to develop, but once it has developed, it lasts. Some dementias are reversible, some are static, and some are progressive. Alzheimer's is always progressive. A sudden apoplectic onset is not typical of early Alzheimer's disease. Neither are seizures, impairment of consciousness, or a suddenly changed gait.

Once you have made a list of symptoms, you should have the patient examined by a competent physician. A clinical evaluation should include a complete history (taken from both the patient and other informants), a physical and neurological examination, and neuropsychologic testing. It is important for the physician to rule out certain reversible conditions by doing a routine blood test. Such conditions include metabolic dysfunctions (like thyroid abnormalities), pernicious anemia, nutritional inadequacies (like deficiencies of B_1 or B_{12}), infectious diseases (like syphilis or AIDS), and neoplastic disorders (like cancer or nonmalignant tumors). Diseases such as Parkinson's and diabetes should also be checked out, and kidney problems should be investigated.

A CT scan of the head and an MRI would rule out such causes as a tumor, a stroke, or excess fluid. They might show that the hippocampus has shrunk significantly. Such shrinkage could indicate the presence of Alzheimer's disease, since the hippocampus is a memory-related center of the brain. However, it would not rule out psychiatric disorders, which should also be explored since clinical depression or a variety of drugs can mimic some of the early symptoms of Alzheimer's disease. Proper treatment of reversible conditions will make the symptoms disappear.

Is the patient suffering from Alzheimer's or from what is commonly called "dementia"? You will no doubt have been told by the doctors you have visited. Technically, what is usually referred to as "Alzheimer's" is called "dementia of the Alzheimer's type," and is one type of dementia among many. However, most people refer to it simply as "Alzheimer's," and consider "dementia" to be slightly different. In this book, I refer to "Alzheimer's/dementia" or just simply "dementia" to acknowledge those commonly held interpretations. No matter what you call it, the disease can be incredibly frustrating for those around the patient, especially since its insidious onset creates doubts and confusion in the caregiver's mind.

By eliminating doubt and confirming the existence of this cruel progressive disease, you are struggling to accept a difficult reality. Part of the difficulty is accepting the fact that your loved one is already at least in the mild stages of the disease. As someone in my support group said of her husband: "He's here, but then again he's not." It will help if you understand what to expect. A neurologist is the most qualified professional you should consult in this area, even if you have seen other doctors. Seek out one who is forthright, compassionate, and is willing to take the time to really talk to you.

Some facts that your neurologist might share with you include the following: Alzheimer's is a neurological condition that causes a deficiency in thinking and remembering. It is the most common cause of dementia. It's named after Alois Alzheimer who identified it in 1906. The actual cause of the disease is unknown, but neuritic plaques, like sticky globs of protein on the outsides of nerve cells, are specifically implicated in Alzheimer's. They are not part of normal aging, and are in greater concentrations in the brains of Alzheimer's patients than in normal older people. Most current research has concentrated on amyloid, a protein that forms these plaques.

Some research has concluded that the sticky amyloid plaque may be the brain's way of protecting itself from the disease, which might be a result of damage to the energy-producing bodies within every cell. This damage could be a result of toxic free radicals that mutated cells cannot destroy.

Different research indicates that the symptoms of Alzheimer's result from the death of nerve cells in the brain. No one knows why they die, and scientists are studying genetic and environmental factors as well as viruses and infectious proteins as potential culprits.

Current research includes the study of abnormal tau protein that makes up the brain tangles that are also characteristic of the disease. Tau normally binds to microtubules, which are the chemical equivalent of train tracks in a cell. Tau is like the ties that connect the tracks. If tau isn't working properly, the microtubules in the brain collapse or tangle together and can't function properly.

Other research is currently concentrating on abnormally lowered glucose utilization in the aging brain. There are new theories and new studies published every week. Newspapers, magazines, medical journals, and TV updates will keep you posted on the latest. Some studies are more reliable than others, so check out the sources.

At this point, there is no definite cure and several types of the disease have been identified, so no one cure will work for all types. Research on dementia is like cancer research because it has to deal with different brain abnormalities that end up producing similar symptoms. The abnormalities range from the abnormal proteins and neurofibrillary tangles already mentioned to concentrations of aluminum. (Incidentally, such concentrations are an aftereffect of the disease, rather than a cause. So you don't have to throw out your favorite pot after all!)

At least four million people in the United States are affected by Alzheimer's disease. Many have the disease but don't seek medical attention. Most cases occur after age sixty, but some people are affected in their forties and fifties. The Alzheimer's Association quotes studies that indicate that 10 percent of people over sixty-five are afflicted. The incidence increases with advancing age to the point where nearly 50 percent of those over eighty-five could have the disease. All segments of the population are affected, with no regard to race or socioeconomic status. Complications of Alzheimer's disease make it the fourth leading cause of death among the elderly in the U.S., claiming 100,000 people annually and costing an estimated $100 billion a year. Your own personal costs will be high, not only financially but emotionally. That is why it is important to line up support on every possible level.

So many people jokingly say that they must have Alzheimer's when they forget things. But it is no joke, and one worries about the possibility of being diagnosed with this malady. I once heard the following guide to see whether or not you have Alzheimer's: If you don't remember where you put your keys, that's not Alzheimer's, but if you are holding your keys in your hand and don't know what they're for, that's cause for concern.

There are specific symptoms that should alert you to the need for a neurological evaluation, even though not everybody experiences all of the symptoms. Some telltale cues of growing cognitive deficits are:

- memory impairment, especially of recently received information (long-term memory continues to function for a longer period of time)
- inability to learn new things
- greater difficulty in performing routine activities
- impaired judgment (refusing to wear a jacket on a cold winter day, for example)
- impaired abstract thinking (inability to distinguish between a chair and a desk, for example)
- impaired spatial concepts (being disoriented and getting lost, for example)
- aphasia (inability to both understand language and produce words correctly)
- agnosia (inability to recognize people, objects, or sounds)
- apraxia (having difficulty moving in a controlled way, such as holding utensils, or using the bathroom. This difficulty is not connected to any limb weakness.)

There are some symptoms that, at first, are not significant enough to give cause for alarm. They are diminished number skills, dwindling ability to write, and personality changes. So when you look back to those times when you couldn't understand your loved one's moodiness or why the checks bounced, you can be more forgiving, as well as sad. Now you know this was just the beginning of a disease over which he/she had no control.

Reference books on the disease outline five stages of Alzheimer's. It can take many years to reach the final stages. As stated before, if the onset is sudden and the progress swift, it's not Alzheimer's. A major illness can trigger a cluster of symptoms. Not every person goes through all the phases in the same way, but you can count on seeing the same general deterioration. The five stages can be summed up as follows:

1. Early Confusion, which may be indicated by:
   — forgetfulness and general confusion
   — slower responses
   — problems communicating
   — personality changes
   — hallucinations and delusions
   — denial of these problems
   — depression and anxiety
2. Advanced Confusion, which may be indicated by:
   — more obvious memory loss
   — greater difficulty in making decisions
   — inability to manage finances properly
   — total denial that there is a problem
   — loss of time and space orientation, making driving a hazard
   — self-absorption and depression
   — greater need of assistance and supervision
3. Early Dementia, which may be indicated by:
   — needing hands-on care
   — needing help in expressing oneself
   — total inability to drive
   — very defensive behavior that leads to making up absurd explanations
   — remembering things that never happened
   — strong emotional reactions, such as crying spells and sudden mood swings, with no apparent provocation
   — good days and bad days with varying memory lapses
   — inability to do things in a logical sequential manner, such as the proper order of dressing
   — needing the feeling of independence, encouraged by the caregiver's helping only when absolutely necessary
   — being overwhelmed by simple decisions
   — social withdrawal

4. Middle Dementia, which may be indicated by:
   — some incontinence
   — greater agitation and hostility
   — delusions expressing irrational fears
   — erratic sleeping
   — repetitive behavior, such as folding and unfolding clothes
   — difficulty moving and coordinating
   — loss of touch with real events and experiences
   — inability to recognize people, even loved ones
   — lack of awareness of location or time (including what year it is)
   — tendency to roam and get lost

At this point, the caregiver feels lonely and isolated. The patient's lack of recognition and communication is crushing. The physical demands of washing, dressing, and attending to the patient's every need are exhausting. The caregiver needs love and support and must figure out how to get relief.

5. Late Dementia, which has been called "the long good-bye" or "the unending death." Both the caregiver and the patient need to touch and listen in order to stay emotionally connected during this phase. This stage may be indicated by:
   — incontinence
   — inability to walk unaided
   — difficulty chewing and swallowing
   — need for constant supervision and assistance
   — stupor leading to coma or death

Knowing the stages of the disease gives one a greater sense of urgency to find a cure. In some cases, drug treatment can slow down the deterioration, but, at this point in time, nothing will completely stop the progress of the disease.

In some twenty controlled double-blind placebo* studies, choline and lecithin were studied to see how they might improve memory and cognitive function. Unfortunately, they did not seem to improve the patients' condition. However, some people still

---

* In a double-blind study, some of the participants are given a placebo—a "dummy pill"—instead of the medication being tested. Neither the patients nor the researchers know whether a particular patient is getting the trial drug or the placebo until after the study.

believe in them. That's because it seems to make sense that lecithin, for one, would be helpful. Here's why: There is a neurotransmitter in the brain called acetylcholine that decreases in Alzheimer's disease because the cells that make it are dying. A logical conclusion would be that this destruction is related to the memory problems experienced by Alzheimer patients. It would seem that anything that can make acetylcholine in the body would improve the symptoms. Lecithin can be used by the body as a raw material to make acetylcholine. Therefore, you'd expect lecithin, readily available in health food stores, to be a cure. Such is not the case: Approximately twenty studies of the use of lecithin as a treatment of Alzheimer's disease showed that it was no more effective than a placebo (but it did seem to help Newton, whereas ginkgo biloba seemed to make him more confused).

There was a well-publicized study favoring the use of ginkgo biloba as a successful treatment for Alzheimer's. This study concluded that the ginkgo extract used had a small but measurable effect on the symptoms of Alzheimer's disease, and appeared relatively safe. Unfortunately, the ginkgo biloba used in the study was a particular extract, prepared in a specific way, and not the kind routinely found on health food store shelves in the United States. Maybe it can be tracked down, if you think it's worth the effort.

Whereas choline and lecithin were administered to try to increase the production of acetylcholine, other drugs are used to try to prevent its breakdown. Ask your doctor about the advisability of prescribing Aricept (donepezil HCl), Cognex (tacrine), or Exelon (rivastigmine). Since these drugs depend on a fairly intact system of neurons and connections, they can usually be of significant benefit to certain patients with moderate dementia, but may also be of some benefit to patients with advanced dementia. While these products are not a cure, they can stabilize cognitive function for an extended period of time.

The FDA regularly reviews drugs that slow the breakdown of acetylcholine within the brain. These drugs have been of some benefit in treating symptoms of Alzheimer's during carefully controlled clinical trials. The FDA is currently considering approval of one called galantamine. We shall see.

It was thought by some doctors that a class of drugs called vasodilators might help by expanding constricted blood vessels in the brain. Some research concluded that vasodilators were more effective in increasing cerebral blood flow in Alzheimer's patients than in normal persons of the same age, but vasodilators have not proven to be of real benefit in treating the disease.

In epidemiologic research, estrogen, antioxidants, and anti-inflammatory agents have been shown to decrease the damage to neurons by slowing down oxidation. Oxidation causes the degeneration of nerve cells. Check with your physician concerning the advisability of trying ginkgo, vitamin E, B_{12}, estrogen, or even lecithin.

Some drugs help some people some of the time, but not everyone responds the same way to each drug. There are various side effects. Cell therapy offers hope, but it is a solution that is in the distant future. That research is in its infancy. Neuronal transplants also hold a promise for the future, but they are still in the research stage.

What does alternative medicine offer? Americans spend billions of dollars on herbal remedies of all kinds. These herbs may be effective, but the treatments have been largely untested scientifically with double-blind studies. The individual concentrations of naturally occurring chemicals in an herbal preparation can vary from brand to brand, or even from one batch to another. These remedies are natural drugs, but drugs nonetheless. (A drug is defined as any substance that we introduce into our bodies in order to alter the body's physiology or function in any way.) Just because a product can be bought without a prescription doesn't mean it shouldn't be regarded as a drug and treated with care. Therefore, these herbal remedies must not be used haphazardly. It is important to verify the quality of the natural remedy you choose.

You must also watch for adverse interactions with other drugs. For example, did you know that ginkgo biloba taken with aspirin may cause unwanted bleeding? Aspirin can have the same inter-action with vitamin E, which is a blood thinner. No matter what you and your physician decide to try, be sure that you finish with one trial before attempting another. When any drug is administered, it usually takes a number of weeks to see results, if there are any. But if you see negative results, don't wait more than two weeks to discontinue the product in question.

In any case, please realize that it's difficult to get a complete pic-ture with only one patient—yours. You are the one who has to deal with the hourly symptoms, and your observations are valid for your situation. However, researchers can't come to a general conclusion without doing a controlled double-blind trial where a potential treat-ment is tested on many people.

One study provides some evidence that vitamin E may be beneficial to Alzheimer patients. But it was a dose of 2000 IU a day that was administered. Such a large dose should never be taken without close medical supervision.

There are commercials on the radio and TV inviting people with memory problems to participate in drug research studies. Should your loved one participate? First of all, only someone at the begin-ning of the disease is eligible. And one must understand the poten-tial risks. There is no guarantee of positive results; the treatment under trial may be ineffective. There may be an additional letdown when there is no significant improvement, if not a worsening of the condition. Besides, a participant cannot be told whether he/she is receiving a placebo (which is not effective) used for the control group. Nonetheless, nothing ventured, nothing gained—you might want to give it a try. At least you can feel the knowledge gained from the trial will be helpful to future generations.

Speaking of future generations, the children of someone with a dementing illness will no doubt be dealing with nagging doubts about inheriting the disease. In my interview with Dr. Marc L. Gordon, I learned that only a small number of families have the gene muta-tion that will be passed on to the next generation. Most Alzheimer cases are "sporadic," occurring here and there, with no clear trait transmitted to children. It is a small minority of Alzheimer patients that have a familial disease. Of course, if you don't have to worry about familial Alzheimer's, we can all worry about sporadic Alzheimer's.

There are some possible preventative treatments. They include postmenopausal estrogen replacement, nonsteroidal anti-inflammatory drugs, vitamin E, and selegiline (Deprenyl). Any of these should be discussed thoroughly with a knowledgeable physician, and the possible side effects should be considered.

As you can see, the diagnosis of Alzheimer's disease announces, without a doubt, the beginning of a life-altering upheaval. Treatments may or may not be effective, even temporarily. Deterioration will continue. You, the caregiver, are now entering a parallel world you never really knew about. You may be tempted by quacks. You will be frightened, isolated, angry, and sad—sometimes all at once. You must remember that there are many others in the same boat as you. Once you find them and learn more and more coping techniques, you will come out of this long twilight. One day, believe me, you will be concerned about ordinary trivia once again.

CHECKLIST

❏ Keep a log of symptoms you think might indicate Alzheimer's disease or dementia.

❏ Make an appointment with your loved one's family physician. Then take him/her to a neurologist.

❏ Contact the Alzheimer's Association for further information and future resources.

❏ Visit your library or bookstore.

❏ Go online, with help if necessary. (Use the information in the resources section at the end of the book as a guide.)

❏ Explore the possibility of participation in a research study.

❏ Look for articles in newspapers and magazines that will inform you of the latest research.

❏ After diagnosis, start making appropriate financial and legal decisions (see chapter 6).

ADDITIONAL READING ABOUT
THE DISEASE AND ITS TREATMENT

Aronson, Miriam, and Robert N. Butler. *Understanding Alzheimer's Disease.* New York: Charles Scribner's Sons, 1998.

Gold, Susan Dudley. *Alzheimer's Disease.* Parsippany, N.J.: Crestwood House, 1996.

Gruetzner, Howard. *Alzheimer's—The Complete Guide for Families and Loved Ones.* New York: John Wiley and Sons, 1997.

Hinnefeld, Joyce. *Everything You Need to Know When Someone You Love Has Alzheimer's Disease.* New York: Rosen Publishing Group, 1994.

Larkin, Marilyn. *When Someone You Love Has Alzheimer's.* New York: Dell, 1995.

McGowin, Dianna Friel. *Living in the Labyrinth.* New York: Bantam Doubleday Dell, 1993.

Nelson, James, and Hilde Lindemann. *Alzheimer's: Answers to Hard Questions for Families.* New York: Bantam Doubleday Dell, 1996.

CHAPTER 2

Effects
of the Disease/
How to Survive

Chapter 1 prepares you for what to expect. Now you need to know how to handle the symptoms. Handling the symptoms means, first, doing as much as possible to keep the patient calm and cooperative while taking proper care of him/her. Second, it means taking care of yourself, both emotionally and physically. Dr. David Narov, a psychologist in Forest Hills, New York, stressed the fact that it's not good to become isolated or overly tense. Therefore, it will help if you develop a mantra that you can repeat to yourself when you are about to lose your cool. "It's a short circuit in the brain," for example, will remind you that the patient has no control over his/her brain's deterioration and isn't doing anything intentionally. Nagging won't help. Everything you do with the brain-impaired person will take more than twice as long as you think it should. You just can't be in a hurry because that will lead to frustration for both of you.

Should you consider giving the patient medication to control emotional instability? That is a question to be answered with the help of your physician. You may not need drugs for a while. In the meantime, the following techniques can be helpful:

Memory Aids

▶ Keep your home neat, and don't rearrange furniture.

▶ "Childproof" your home.

▶ Place labels on cabinets, doors, and boxes to identify contents.

▶ Establish daily routines. Write them out in outline form and place them where needed.

▶ Hang up an erasable bulletin board on which you write the day and date, including the year, and the day's appointments. In this way, when you are asked repeated questions, you can direct the patient to the bulletin board. A calendar will also be helpful, providing you mark off the days.

▶ Write out as much instruction as you can for simple tasks.

▶ Use simple sentences and short explanations whenever possible.

Reality Orientation

▶ Mention the day or time and names of objects and people in conversation.

▶ Avoid talking down to the patient, all the while keeping in mind that his/her thinking ability is reduced to that of a very young child.

▶ Encourage the person with dementia to perform as many independent daily activities as possible. Overlook mismatched socks, etc.

▶ Give clear-cut choices, presenting desirable and undesirable activities. Example: At dinner time, say "Do you want to eat dinner now or pick up the laundry?"

▶ Only correct mistakes when absolutely necessary, and if so, do it gently.

Reminiscence Techniques

You want the patient to focus on what he/she can remember. If the patient is receptive, this will build self-esteem, which can make the patient less depressed and reduce your own sadness. Of course, sometimes reminiscing can bring on sadness, so you should use this technique carefully.

- Ask specific questions about past events.
- Encourage continued talking by asking follow-up questions.
- Encourage talk of past goals and achievements.
- Acknowledge and validate the person's feelings.
- Make few comments, just listen. Overlook the patient's denial of reality.
- Change the topic if the memory seems painful.
- Use sensory cues such as pictures, music, and food.

Anxiety Relievers

- Touching and hugging
- Genuine compliments
- Structured activities
- Repeated schedules
- Simple instructions
- Physical activities, such as walking, gardening, or playing games; daily exercise
- Listening to music
- Respecting fatigue and avoiding more difficult concepts at that time
- Elimination of caffeine (including caffeine in tea and sodas)

Avoid violent TV programs since the disease often robs a person of the ability to distinguish between what is real and what is not. Shut the blinds and drape sheets over mirrors at night to lessen the chance that your loved one will wake up with hallucinations in the middle of the night.

Communication Aids

- Patience
- A relaxed atmosphere, including lack of pressure
- Elimination of distractions, such as TV or radio, when you want to have a conversation
- Asking "yes" or "no" questions if communication is difficult
- Always being very specific
- Using simple words while speaking clearly and slowly

▶ Using flash cards

▶ Acting out an activity

If your loved one stops in mid-sentence, having lost his/her train of thought, repeat exactly what you heard previously, and wait patiently for the completion of the sentence. Be aware of body language and tone of voice to make sense of what the patient can't express verbally. Be sure the eyeglasses and hearing aid work. You can get the patient's attention with a gentle touch or by saying his/her name. If you must repeat something, first try using exactly the same words you used before. That assumes, of course, that you are using very basic sentences.

When it reaches the point where medication is necessary to influence your loved one's behavior, you should try to read up on background information before discussing this option with the doctor. Due to continued research, there are new drugs available constantly. Consider all the facets of a drug's effects: at a time when you desperately need to calm your patient, you might not be focusing on side effects. However, if these side effects make the patient sicker or harder to manage, you will have to change drugs. Do not hesitate to call your doctor to ask for a modification. That is one of the few things over which you have some control. Your library and local bookstore are a source for research and background information about drugs. (See the suggested reading list at the end of this chapter, as well as after chapter 1.)

Medications can sometimes reduce some symptoms of Alzheimer's. Responses vary greatly: a patient can experience anything from definite benefits to no change to a worsening of the symptoms. It is advisable to start at low dosages and increase them slowly. You may want rapid relief, but this method is safer since side effects are more likely to occur at high dosages. Negative side effects will be smaller with smaller amounts of medication. Lower doses also allow the body to adjust gradually. You should never modify the dose yourself. It is crucial to rely on the patient's physician to adjust doses. You can change doctors but should always have only one in charge of psychotropic medication. Sometimes there is an interaction between drugs.

Although minor side effects might be easy to ignore in exchange for a more docile patient, some tranquilizers (neuroleptics or antipsychotics) can create more severe physical symptoms. Tranquilizers can lower blood pressure, create dizziness, and result in a fall. They can cause muscle rigidity, which shows itself as drooling, a shuffling gait, or tremors. Another reaction may cause the patient to feel agitated, unable to sit still or sleep. So, an attempt to help yourself can increase your workload rather than make your life easier. That's why it will help if you have realistic expectations of the medication. Changes, if any, may be moderate.

It is often necessary to hospitalize the patient while verifying drugs and dosages. The best place to do that is in a psychiatric ward. Your loved one might act unacceptably there, becoming either violent or overly withdrawn. It would be painful for you to witness this. For that reason, as well as for general peace of mind, you should be alert to what affects your loved one. Watch for unacceptable behavior not connected to medication. There may be a solution in other environmental factors. For example, I soon discovered that Newton, who was a diabetic, became totally erratic and resistant if he had had even a tiny amount of sugar. So I was extra vigilant to prevent his having any kind of sweets, even the small amount of sugar in a hamburger roll.

Only you, the caregiver, who is constantly with the patient, are in a position to observe any connection between cause and effect. It is really worthwhile keeping some kind of log handy so you can write down possible triggers to unacceptable behavior. When you reread a few pages of the log, a pattern might emerge. You can then present your suspicions to the neurologist. You might get a skeptical reaction. The fact of the matter is that you are the one living with the patient, and therefore you know what the behavioral changes are. Accept the use of medication for the patient as you see fit.

What about medication for you? When you hurt, you cry, but if the crying doesn't stop, you may need medication yourself. The side effects may be negligible, worth some small discomfort in exchange for being less tense. If you have trouble sleeping, though, it may be due as much to exhaustion as to tension. Make getting a decent amount of sleep a priority. Let the dust sit. Don't iron. Go to see your own doctor to discuss possible solutions. As time-consuming as it may be, you must change doctors if your own physician is too busy to listen. A prescription by itself may be inadequate if you need to talk about all the stresses and changes within you.

Your eating habits may have changed. You probably neglect your own nutritional needs in favor of the patient's. You may be losing weight or gaining because you're eating junk food. You know this is not good for you, but you don't care. That, however, will only diminish your ability to help.

Do your utmost to get out of the house by yourself for at least an hour every day. That will clear your mind and make you a better caregiver besides helping you to survive. Thinking of you will enable you to think properly about your loved one who is at times lost in a private vortex. Because the person with dementia is unstable and unreliable, you have to have stability for both of you.

Accept the fact that you cannot halt the progression of the disease. It is normal to cry with the slightest provocation. You are bewildered. Don't reproach yourself. Seek out the few people who are really supportive. You are not dumping. You are replenishing your life energy.

The hardest part of being a helpless witness to the mental deterioration of a loved one is accepting the reality of the situation. However, it is this very acceptance that will make your life less stressful: Once you know what to expect, you can more readily deal with whatever comes up. You won't be as angry at the ill person since you will be less likely to think difficult behavior is his/her fault. That's not to say that you won't become impatient when you see behavior that makes no sense to you. But understanding what's behind this behavior will enable you to tolerate it better.

For your own sanity you ought to read up on the disease as much as you need to. Maybe chapter 1 of this book will be adequate.

If you need more information, take the time. Your day-to-day survival will depend on your getting whatever intellectual, emotional, and physical support you need to function. It's OK to give to yourself. These gifts do not need to be expensive and they do not need to take a lot of time: A fifteen-minute soak in a warm bath will reenergize you for hours. It may seem self-indulgent to take that bath in the middle of the day when the laundry is piling up, but a time-out for yourself is a lot more important than laundry or dirty floors.

There is a high burnout rate in primary caregivers of dementia patients. Being tired is one thing, but being chronically exhausted renders you unable to take proper care of the one who needs the most care: Your judgment is impaired, your fuse is much too short, and you can't give the patient as much as you really want to. So your highest priority must be you. Self-sacrifice is self-defeating.

It is easier said than done to take care of yourself first. You are naturally drawn to your loved one and to all the responsibilities that come with the illness. For that reason, you should structure your day so that it does not slip away in the blink of an eye. Make appointments for yourself as well as for the patient. If you enjoy going to the movies, do it. If you prefer walking, make a date to walk with a friend and keep it. The point is, you need to focus on a specific time when you can remove yourself from the engulfing world of a caregiver.

How can you give yourself the validation, comfort, and encouragement that you need? Maybe you'd be comfortable joining a support group. It doesn't matter whether you like to talk or not. Listening brings comfort, too. A whole new world presents itself when you are in the company of fellow sufferers. That's why there is such a proliferation of support groups of all kinds. Some people need to overcome their reluctance to "hear other people's problems" or talk about private matters. But it is those other people's problems that will show you that you are not alone. Your isolation can swallow you up. Your loved one will benefit as much as you since you will be better equipped to handle all the situations that come up. It's surprising how ignorant I was when I was a solitary caregiver. My support group expanded my vision and actually calmed me. I was able to appreciate humorous or tender moments with Newton much more easily once I realized that I was not alone in being a caregiver.

Where to find the appropriate support group? First contact the Alzheimer's Association in your area. Don't settle for anything that meets too rarely or costs too much. Getting together once a week is not often at all. Way before the next meeting, you'll be ready for renewed support. Persevere in your search for a group. Here are some useful addresses:

▷ U.S. Department of Health and Human Services
Alzheimer's Disease Education and Referral Center
P.O. Box 8250
Silver Spring, MD 20907
(800) 438-4380

▷ American Health Assistance Foundation
15825 Shady Grove, Suite 140
Rockville, MD 20850
(800) 437-2423

▷ National Association of Area Agencies on Aging
927 15th St. NW
Washington, DC 20005
(202) 296-8130

It amazes me that I did not think of contacting such an association for months. I was so dulled by my overwhelming responsibilities and confused by a disease I knew nothing about. Looking for support, I tried all sorts of other avenues that were inadequate at best. Then the light bulb went on when someone casually mentioned the Alzheimer's Association. I wasn't sure they could help me since Newton did not actually have Alzheimer's, but help me they did: They referred me to a weekly group that accepted the caregivers of various dementias, including Alzheimer's disease. The leader, a social worker, was simply wonderful. And I didn't have to pay anything! (You better believe that I make charitable contributions to the Alzheimer's Association regularly.) I really wanted to go back to a meeting within two days. Fortunately, there were other members of the group I could call on for release. They called me too, of course.

You can't develop deep friendships at this point; you're too busy surviving. But these other caregivers become, not your actual soul mates, but "support mates" with whom you share intimate emotional and physical details. You don't have to explain anything to them. You don't have to justify yourself. They just understand. That kind of support is invaluable.

Should you also consider individual counseling? It certainly would not be a luxury, nor would it duplicate or contradict what is happening in a support group. Times of crisis (and this is a crisis bar none) bring out unresolved issues. So this might be the perfect opportunity to examine how you feel about life and family. You can also get much needed individual guidance and support from a counselor. If you choose private counseling, should you go to a social worker, a psychologist, or a psychiatrist? A psychiatrist is a medical doctor who specializes in psychiatry and so is allowed to prescribe medication. If you feel the need for an antidepressant, you will want to see a psychiatrist. Otherwise, a psychologist will do fine if you want to explore deep issues, since a psychologist has a doctorate and is trained extensively in the parameters of human behavior. A social worker must have at least a master's degree and thorough training to become a CSW (certified social worker). Since that takes less time than the other training, social workers charge less for their services than the other two. By the same token, psychiatrists charge the most, since their training takes the most time.

The secret to success is finding someone you can trust. No matter how prestigious someone's degrees are, you won't make progress if you don't feel comfortable confiding in that individual. It is not the therapist who makes you change and grow, it is his/her professional guidance that shows you the way to change yourself. There is something warmly reassuring about knowing that a chunk of time is devoted only to you, your thoughts, your needs, and your goals.

Although your patient's goals have been drastically altered, that does not mean that he/she wouldn't also benefit from some private therapy. In the earlier stages, having a willing and professional ear is a comfort. The therapist can not only support your loved one, but validate his/her feelings. This will give the person with a dementing illness consolation and inner peace, even briefly. That's worth a lot.

Therapy is not cheap. However, it is money well spent. How much money you spend will depend not only on the credentials of your therapist, but also on your income. There are counseling agencies of all kinds, some associated with hospitals. They will use a sliding scale and charge little or nothing to those who can't afford to pay the full fee. That means that you may have to pay something, but it won't take the food off your table.

Everyone has heard jokes about people in therapy for thirty years. Don't worry, you can quit whenever you want. If you were the type to go on "forever," you would already be in therapy. Look in the yellow pages of your phone book under "mental health" or call a local hospital. Your doctor probably can give you the name of a reliable therapist. Or you can ask around, if you feel comfortable doing so. Maybe your health plan provides partial coverage for these services and has a listing of participating providers. If you do not feel at ease with the first counselor you meet, please do not hesitate to find another one. Only if you have changed therapists several times should you begin to wonder what's wrong with you.

You have considered your emotional and psychological needs as well as those of your patient. Now you are ready to tackle the physical challenges that await you. By planning ahead and "dementia proofing" your home, you can considerably lighten your load. The next chapter will guide you on physical techniques.

CHECKLIST

❏ Prepare your home and your routines to make life simpler for both you and the patient.

❏ Read up on medication available to treat Alzheimer's or other dementias.

❏ Do as much research on the disease as you need to. How little or how much is entirely up to you.

❏ Find yourself a doctor who is not too busy to listen.

❏ Communicate your concerns with a supportive doctor. Change doctors if necessary.

❏ Consider the advisability of taking tranquilizers yourself.

❏ Be sure to take proper care of yourself: sleep enough and eat regularly. Avoid junk food.

❏ Schedule regular activities for yourself as well as for your loved one, together and separately.

❏ Join a support group.

❏ Explore individual counseling for you and/or the patient.

SUGGESTED ADDITIONAL READING ABOUT DEALING WITH THE EFFECTS OF THE DISEASE

Anifantakis, Harry. *The Diminished Mind*. Blue Ridge Summit, Pa.: Tab Books, 1991.

Charlesworth, E. A., and R. G. Nathan. *Stress Management*. New York: Ballantine, 1982.

Hodgson, Harriet. *The Alzheimer's Caregiver*. Minnetonka, Minn.: Chronimed Publishing, 1998.

Kushner, Harold S. *When Bad Things Happen to Good People*. New York: Schocken Books, 1989.

Woolfolk, R. L., and P. M. Lehrer. *Principles and Practices of Stress*. New York: Guilford Press, 1989.

CHAPTER 3

How to Help and Get Help for the Patient and for You

Here you are in a situation you never expected to be in. It's like being in a prison without walls, and you don't know how long your sentence is. Your first goal will be to figure out how to handle the various complications as they come up. Your most important goal is to take care of yourself, but you won't realize that right away. That's why there is a separate chapter devoted to your own survival. Most caregivers see themselves as being able to do more than they really can, and over time the burden becomes enormous. It is important not to take on more chores than you can reasonably handle. There are only so many hours in a day, and just doing the minimum gobbles them up.

The first thing to do is enable the patient to be as independent as possible for as long as possible. That means, for example, putting up support rails in the shower or bathtub. If the patient thinks he/she doesn't need them, say you're doing this for your own needs. In the long run, that's true: having those bars will make a tremendous difference. If the patient has something solid to hold on to, he/she will feel more secure and will step into the shower more willingly. Besides, you won't have to worry about a fall as much. You should also have a plastic mat or strips on the floor of the tub. Another vital piece of equipment is a plastic bench to put into the tub. A detachable showerhead attached to a flexible hose comes in very handy, too.

So, now, how do you give a 170-pound person a shower? My own method, which I figured out by trial and error before anyone would tell me the "official" way, is as follows: First run the water and have the patient feel that the temperature is comfortable. Then have him/her step into the tub while holding on to the support rails. Using the flexible hose, wet the buttocks and crotch, then lather and rinse that area. Afterwards, the patient can sit and you can easily wash the rest of the body. If you want to wash his/her hair, do that afterwards. Once the shower is over with, turn off the water, and dry him/her off while the patient is still sitting on the bench. That way, you only have to dry the lower legs, feet, and crotch area out of the tub.

The way most professional caregivers are trained to give a shower is to have the patient sit right away and have him/her lift up one thigh at a time, as though starting to cross his/her legs, and wash and rinse each section at a time.

If your patient is afraid of showers, and wants only baths, I urge you to gradually introduce showers at the beginning of the illness because it's very hard to lift someone out of a tub without help. There are lifts to lower and raise someone, but they're expensive. (Lifting becomes necessary because one day the patient will be unable to cooperate as the dementia progresses.) If all else fails, you can give a sponge bath, but that's harder and less effective. Maybe a portable sitz bath (bidet) would help. In any case, be alert to the danger of electric shock when your ward is in water, and don't allow any electrical appliances to be within reach.

Look in the yellow pages of your phone directory to find the names of surgical supply stores (see also the resources section). They are the most likely to have the equipment you need, and if they don't carry a product, they will guide you to the appropriate supplier. These supply houses also sell raised toilet seats and bars to put around the toilet, so the patients can lower themselves more easily and hoist themselves up as well. That seems to require little concentration, and enables patients to use the toilet on their own for quite a while. What does seem to require concentration is proper use of the toilet paper. You must help in that.

You must help *yourself* whenever possible, also. Therefore, start buying your loved one pull-on pants and shirts so no one will have to fumble with buttons and zippers. Slacks are more practical than skirts. There are occasions when you can give these items as gifts. You can always create an opportunity. In addition, an ID bracelet is crucial. You can get one from a mail-order house or in a drug store. You might also want to enroll your loved one in the Safe Return Program ([800] 272-3900). To prevent the patient from leaving home to begin with, put a latch at the top of the door jamb. Even a hook and eye can keep the person in since he/she won't look up and try to figure out how to open the door.

As the deterioration proceeds, you have to adjust. Hang up a simple bulletin board or an erasable board in the kitchen or an area where you often sit. Write down the day's appointments so both you and the patient can refer to the list as often as needed. You can also use this board to make a check-off chart listing necessary medications. (There is a medication chart for this purpose in the resources section.) That way, you will avoid over- or undermedicating the patient.

Although there are no shortcuts to administering medication, you can simplify the way prescriptions are filled: work out a system with your local pharmacist that will make it unnecessary for you to go to the pharmacy. A tip to the delivery person is well worth the energy you save. You can have maintenance drugs delivered by mail, along with things like diabetic supplies. Mail-order drugs are more likely to be covered by drug insurance and are cheaper than store-bought ones. It may take time to set things up, but you will then save a lot more precious time in the long run.

There are other time- and energy-saving aids to consider. They include a swiveling car seat cushion so the patient can get out more easily, large decals to put on glass doors that otherwise appear open, and adhesive tape for floor mats or throw rugs so they won't slip. If possible, you should remove the floor mats altogether because they will interfere with a shuffling gait.

Keep anything potentially dangerous out of reach, from guns to matches. Childproof the stove and cabinet doors. Also remember that, as good judgment disappears, your loved one may try to eat pebbles or plastic fruits.

The person with dementia will certainly not always be cooperative. You will therefore have many opportunities to practice self-control. Since intense light encourages greater agitation, use soft lights wherever possible. Use a quiet voice. At times, you might still shout despite yourself. It's when you want to be physical and hit the person that you must walk out of the room. The sad fact is that your emotional outbursts will not help the situation, and won't even relieve you of tension, since you will feel guilty for having been nasty. So remind yourself often that this person in front of you is no longer the one you knew, and that he/she just can't help being the way he/she is.

Most adults do not relish the idea of wearing diapers. That's probably why the manufacturers diplomatically call them "adult briefs." After two or three accidents, though, it's time to adopt this option. I suggest telling rather than asking. Point out that, for both your sakes, it would be a big help if the patient wore these, so you wouldn't have to change every single item of clothing, from undershirt to socks, whenever it isn't possible to "make it in time." You could start putting these "briefs" on for nighttime. We tried cotton briefs with plastic inner liners early on, but they weren't enough. Finally, we both accepted reality. Like with anything in life, the way one person handles the situation affects the way the other reacts. It was incredibly painful for both of us the first time I put one of those "briefs" on him. He knew.

To protect your mattress, place an old shower curtain or felt-backed tablecloth under the sheet. To protect the sheet and reduce your laundry load, place plastic-backed pads on top of the sheet.

They can be found with the adult diapers in supermarkets as well as in drug stores.

All these aids cost money. They are not considered "durable medical equipment" by Medicare, and I gave up trying to get refunds—I just wasted my time, and that of the doctor who was willing to testify to the necessity of the toilet bars, and so on. You might find some used equipment listed in the classified ads of local papers. Some volunteer ambulance corps lend out supplies. If you must borrow money to buy the right equipment, it is well worth it. It will spare you physically and emotionally.

One piece of equipment that is likely not to be of much help is a walker: using a walker requires the conscious coordination of several movements in sequence. That makes it hard for a person with dementia to use. A wheelchair might come in handy at some point, and can be obtained through Medicare if a doctor certifies that the patient needs it at all times. So it isn't necessary to work on that right away. Medicaid supplies a greater variety of help, both with equipment and staff. If the patient is eligible for Medicaid, you will be told what helpers and aids are available (see chapter 6).

If you have a staircase in your home, two handrails will eventually save hours of stressful effort to get the patient upstairs. Since many dementia sufferers are afraid of falling, they cling to the one railing, and won't let go. There are also electrical moving rails equipped with seats, but they really cost a lot. There may be used ones for sale in the paper. Or you could simply set up a bedroom on the ground floor, if a bathroom is handy. (It's easier to bring the patient up the stairs than it is to build a shower in the kitchen.)

There is equipment that will lift a patient from a bed to a wheelchair, but there is nothing out there to pick someone up from the floor. Although 911 will respond and help pick someone off the floor, you really can't rely on that any more than you can rely on good neighbors or friends to help time and again. When you feel trapped and helpless, that's your signal to get hired help on a regular basis: You must be willing to hire someone to come on a daily basis, to hire a live-in aide, or to place your charge in a nursing home. All three choices require a lot of thinking and emotional as well as physical adjusting.

If you choose to hire someone to come in for a certain number of hours each day, that person can be a tremendous help with laundry, shopping, and especially caregiving. But if you need extra help at the wrong time of day, or in the middle of the night, you're stuck. People with Alzheimer's don't always sleep for long, and they tend to wander, physically as well as mentally. They can also make a lot of noise. You might then prefer a live-in helper, who will leave you on your own only on days off. At this stage of exhaustion, loss of privacy seems surprisingly unimportant. If the patient is in a nursing home, you have none of those decisions to make, but there are other concerns that are addressed in chapter 5. At this point, the question is, How do you find a good helper?

If you are unable to administer a medical necessity to your loved one, such as giving injections or changing dressings, you are entitled through Medicare to have a visiting nurse come to attend to those needs. Once a nurse comes, you may be entitled to other support services for a few hours a day, a few days a week. The nurse determines what is needed.

If you aren't eligible for such service, you will need to turn to other options. There are fine placement agencies that screen and train their staff before sending them out to people's homes. Unfortunately, you have to pay a lot for such helpers. Sometimes you may not be satisfied with a particular aide, and the agency may be able to send you someone else who will be more to your liking. To check out an agency, find out what kind of accreditation it has, and ask for several references. Check out those references thoroughly. What kind of questions should you ask? Start off by finding out exactly what the aide did to help the patient. Listen very carefully to the tone of voice as well as the words you hear. Here's a final query that eliminates lingering doubts: "Would I be making a mistake if I used this placement agency (or this aide)?" Ask the agency personnel contact how they check out their employees. There have been news stories about caretakers with criminal records.

In any case, remove all articles of value that are easy to tuck away. That includes jewelry in a drawer. Better to be safe than sorry. I've heard too many tales of thievery not to believe that it happens often. You might want to open a safety deposit box with someone you trust and put your valuables away. If you can spare the space, change the simple doorknob of a chosen room to one that locks, and keep the door locked. Hold the key on you or keep it well hidden. If an entire room can't be locked up, try a closet or a file cabinet with a lock. You want to keep out anyone who doesn't belong—including the patient—who could make a real mess of things. If you remove temptation, you also remove potential problems, and you've got enough of those.

What if you have ruled out a placement agency, and are not eligible for any other substantial support? How can you find an individual to help? Ask around. Look in your local paper, the supermarket bulletin board, or a senior center. You can also place your own ad in the newspaper, specifying exactly the kind of help you are seeking. Research references very carefully and listen to your gut reaction. Draw up a list of questions you would like to ask the people given as a reference. You should check out at least three references. You could inquire about the duties the caregiver performed, about his/her willingness to volunteer help, his/her attitude toward the patient and toward the other family members, and, of course, about that person's honesty. Also ask why he/she is no longer working there.

When you interview your potential helper, try to do it with the patient present. You want them to get along, and you want to eliminate possible unpleasant surprises. Verify that the aide knows enough English to communicate successfully with your loved one. I drew up a list of seven questions after letting my first aide go. They included: "How do you help someone out of a car when he can't get out on his own?" "How do you give a shower?" "How can you pick up my heavy husband from the floor?" I also presented some tough situations I had experienced and asked how she would handle them.

It will avoid future problems if you come to a clear understanding of the specific duties you want performed. Writing them down will leave no room for doubt. Be realistic, but don't hesitate to demand that your helper actually help rather than watch TV. I won't deny that every worker needs a break. However, I refused to hire the woman who told me she would not do laundry or vacuum while my husband was sleeping for hours. She wanted to be inactive while I did the work, and my burden wouldn't have been lightened by much.

How much do you pay? Is minimum wage enough? That depends on your area, the person's experience, and your needs. Here's the big problem: Who wants to do this kind of work? It might be an angel on earth—and there really are some around. However, far too often it is someone who can't find another type of job: with no high school diploma or no marketable skills, or with illegal immigrant status, this person is desperate for any job. Although you might also be desperate for relief at the time you hire someone, keep in mind that it is much easier to hire than to fire. Go slowly and be thorough. Be clear as to what you want done. I discussed details with the second helper I hired, having learned the hard way that it was necessary to do so. Mind you, that did not insure success: that helper left me stranded while Newton was on his long deathbed, after having said some unthinkably cruel things to me. Yes, I had checked her out, but not enough, and I hadn't listened to my sixth sense that told me there was something not quite right about her references. So I joined the legions of family members who seek good help and do not always find it, or think they have reliable people only to have those people leave unexpectedly.

Before you hire anyone, you should also consult a tax professional about how to handle Social Security, withholding tax, and unemployment insurance. With the additional paperwork comes greater peace of mind. Of course, we all know of friends who did not bother with Social Security for their hired help. This is a decision you must make for yourself. Just be aware of the possible consequences of whatever you decide.

Should you have a family member or close friend helping you, there would be no Social Security concerns. But as the saying goes, there's no such thing as free lunch. Valued relationships, with friends or family, can be strained to the limit under these circumstances. You might be better off calling on these good people only in a crisis. You can be sure you will have occasion to ask for their help. They can act as a brief transition between your going it alone and paying for help. It's not a good idea to be a martyr. Waiting until you're completely frazzled won't help anybody.

If you decide to keep your loved one out of an institutional setting, you probably need outside help even if it's not every day. There are agencies for the aging paid for with our taxes. Look for them in the blue pages of your phone book under "senior" or "aging" categories (also see the resources section). If you can't find help on your own, call your local government representative's office. The staff can probably give you some leads.

What kind of occasional help is out there, for little or no money? Meals-on-Wheels will feed the sick person, not you, but that relieves you of the responsibility of some of the cooking. You can arrange for low-cost transportation that will take you along as your ward's helper. You can get a little rest while someone else does the driving. Take advantage of every possible form of assistance, even if it's not much. I accepted help with laundry at $1.00 an hour, with the balance subsidized by government agencies. Too bad it was only for two hours, every other week! Still, I signed up for it, figuring it was at least something. I went through the interview in my home. I waited patiently until my turn came a few weeks later. Then the laundry helper came, washed and dried a fraction of what I had to do every day, and later complained to her supervisor that there was so much laundry, I must have been giving her someone else's to do also! When her supervisor, the social worker, called to tell me this, I just lost it. I screamed at her, used some crude language, hung up, and cried. I decided to hire my own help. It turned out to be a kind acquaintance who has since become a friend. She was gracious enough to accept payment for something she would gladly have done for free: She understood that I didn't want to impose, and she protected my fragile pride. She even did ironing!

You will find that not all the relief offered is effective. But you really should look into every possibility. There is respite care on different levels. Some programs will send a volunteer to read to the patient or play music a mere once a month, while others will come to pick up the sick one and take him/her to a daytime facility more than once a week. Some are very reasonable, some are expensive. Some are well run, while some are slapped together in dingy quarters. Although it takes time and energy to investigate all the possibilities, it pays off in the long run. An hour here or there can allow you to take a bath or a nap, or just get out of the house.

One day, I came home at five o'clock in the evening after driving my husband to several medical visits. It was time to prepare supper. I was exhausted, and the thought of cooking just paralyzed me. That's when I decided I needed cooking help. I called local senior centers, figuring there would be some retiree who enjoyed cooking and would want to make some pocket money. There was no such person available. However, the daughter of one of the secretaries in a senior center was interested in trying it out. She was a savior. In only two hours once a week, she made large quantities of delicious food that I froze in meal-sized portions. I always had something to heat up and serve, and I didn't mind shopping for the ingredients.

Someone else might crave relief in a different category. Whatever your greatest burden, you can figure out a way to lighten your load. It pays to give it some thought. You don't have to spend a lot. Besides, if you've been saving for a rainy day, it's pouring. Save *yourself*, don't worry about the money: that's cheaper than your falling sick. Exhaustion depletes your immune system.

What if you should need a few days off? One form of respite care found in many localities is offered by nursing homes (the yellow pages may also call them "homes for the aged"). They will house your loved one for a limited time, be it a week or a few days. You can take a vacation or attend an important family function. Their rates are surprisingly reasonable. They can administer medication and take adequate care of the patient. If the setting isn't perfect, you know that it's only temporary. How can you find such a place? Make some phone calls, ask other caregivers, call nursing homes directly. Whenever someone tells you he/she can't do something you need done, always ask whether he/she knows someone who can. You can gather a lot of information that way.

No matter what, don't give up. If it all seems too much to handle, take a shower, go out for a few minutes, cuddle with your loved one, and remember that tomorrow always brings new possibilities and insights.

CHECKLIST

☐ Set up your bathtub and shower with safety strips, flexible hose, handrails securely fastened to the wall, and a plastic shower bench to sit on.

☐ Install a raised toilet seat and standing bars connected to the toilet bowl.

☐ Be sure there are two railings along any steps the patient will need to use.

☐ Buy pull-on pants with an elastic waist and pullover tops as well as extra underwear and a supply of "adult briefs."

☐ Protect the bedding with a plasticized cover.

☐ Take fifteen minutes just for yourself every day, no matter what responsibilities await you.

☐ Contact the Alzheimer's Association and ask them to send you materials.

☐ Draw up a list of what you need help with the most. Keep that list on hand so you can get appropriate help.

☐ Evaluate whether or not you want to call on family and friends for help rather than paying someone.

☐ Ask around ahead of time about aides and keep names and numbers for future reference.

☐ Check with an accountant concerning procedures for handling payroll taxes.

❑ Look through the blue pages of your phone book to locate senior citizen services. Call each one to find out what relief they can offer you, including day care facilities.

**ADDITIONAL READING
FOR GIVING AND GETTING HELP**

Alzheimer's Association publications. Call (800) 272-3900 to order.

Mace, Nancy L., and Peter V. Rabins. *The 36-Hour Day.* Baltimore: Johns Hopkins University Press, 1999.

Visiting Nurse Association of America (VNAA). *Caregiver's Handbook.* New York: DK Publishing, 1998.

CHAPTER 4

Sources
of Strength
and Courage

The entertainment media have given us an idealized version of family life. In reality, however, things just don't work out that way. If unresolved issues create unpleasant undercurrents at gatherings such as Thanksgiving, they really come to the surface during a family crisis. Having a family member stricken with dementia, be it Alzheimer's or another type, certainly qualifies as a crisis.

Research indicates that most family members are supportive, but many of them are uncertain about what to do. If they are unsupportive, it is that fact that is most upsetting to a caregiver. One appreciates the concern and assistance of distant family members, but one expects the support of children or siblings. Grown children may be adults, but in their hearts they are still a parent's baby. That is why it can be so difficult for some healthy spouse caregivers to get adequate help from the child of a person with dementia. One would think that a child who loves his stricken parent would want to do as much as possible for him/her. If the loving caregiver is overwhelmed, shouldn't a child want to shoulder some of the burden? The answers are far too often in the negative. Old sibling rivalry and just plain fear take over. No matter how concerned a child may be, he/she often has trouble dealing with the helplessness of seeing a parent deteriorate mentally. That leaves the care-giver to handle the daily mini-crises that arise once a person's dementia has reached a more advanced stage. People in the early stages of the disease present challenges that are very different: They are frightened and puzzled, and often in denial. They may or may not be willing to cooperate with advance planning.

People in support groups aren't representative of all caregivers, but those in my group shared a number of frustrations concerning family members. Many tears were shed by mothers whose children had virtually abandoned them and the stricken father. The result-ing hurt and isolation made it difficult to face each day. The great-est frustration was being unable to comprehend how an apparently loving child could turn his back on you at a time of such obvious need. Some children called once a week and kept the conversation short and superficial, while others didn't call at all. This is not to say that there aren't children who come running to help. They are the ones interviewed in chapter 9. We are dealing here with the agony suffered by the abandoned spouse caregiver.

What about the impaired person's siblings? If they can, they will be more likely to respond. However, their own health and location may make direct assistance impossible. Although they may phone fairly frequently and share some of the caregiver's feelings, they too may be more threatened by the illness than moved to come to the rescue. Their overriding concern, consciously or unconsciously, is whether or not they will be stricken next. Not everyone can deal with the mental deterioration of a stranger, let alone that of a beloved family member. The caregiver therefore has to work hard at being understanding at the very time when he/she desper-ately *needs* understanding.

Not everyone has siblings available. So, the next step is turning to friends. Even long-time friends also cannot always deal with the situation. It can come as a shock when good friends just turn their backs. They also feel threatened and upset. They don't even have family obligations to push them to be helpful. Nonetheless, since friends are chosen and cultivated rather than born, their lack of support is equally devastating. They just may not want to deal with the limitations of a handicapped person in their midst. They would therefore prefer not to go out with you anymore, or even visit.

Since people are uncomfortable with a person with dementia, they become uncomfortable with the caregiver also. It's a matter of ignorance. They don't know what to do with this person who is no longer the one they knew. Instead of asking questions so they can deal with it, they choose to ignore the situation. That is painful for everyone, but the truth is that those who have not been touched by a dementing illness really don't know what to say, or even whether they should say anything. They certainly don't know what to do.

There are, of course, friends who are able to deal with the situation and who come through more than you dreamed possible. Those are the people to cherish, even after the nightmare is over. However, this does not mean that you completely eliminate from your life those who just couldn't be available for you. Forgiveness is therapeutic. If you reach out to those who don't know how to reach out to you, you may get some heartwarming results.

In the meantime, consider joining a support group, providing that won't make you too uncomfortable. If you do join such a group, you will make friends out of strangers among the group's members. It beats talking to strangers in the supermarket and pouring your heart out unexpectedly while you're standing on line. You will be able to speak guilt-free to the members of a support group. You will not feel embarrassed after you've finished. With these fellow caregivers, you can engage in such mundane activities as going out to lunch. They understand you and you understand them. This is not just a case of making lemonade when life hands you lemons; it's a case of expanding your horizons while overcoming adversity.

Overcoming adversity means that the caregiver's inner resources now must be pushed to the limit. There are a variety of activities one can participate in alone or with a mentally handicapped person. Think simple. Watching a movie on television while sitting close to your loved one will not only make the time pass and temporarily remove you from reality, it will also create a new closeness. If the afflicted person is capable of taking a walk, that should become a scheduled daily activity. You will be refreshed by the change of scenery. Your mood will be improved by physical activity even if you must walk slowly. You can also take folding chairs and sit outside or go to a mall and watch the world go by. As you can see, small treats do not require a great deal of effort.

Having a pet requires more effort, especially at the beginning. If you adopt an older pet, the odds are it has been housebroken and you wouldn't have to worry about that aspect of pet ownership. Why take in another mouth to feed? Because a pet usually accepts its owner unconditionally. In addition, the owner is often soothed by petting the animal and sensing its presence.

Researchers have studied the effect that animals have on the well-being of humans across a life cycle. The results are enlightening: dogs, cats, or even ferrets can supply comfort and reduce feelings of loneliness during stressful times. They also provide an opportunity to be nurturing, something an Alzheimer's/dementia patient has little opportunity to do. Having a family pet enhances your quality of life. It gives you a purpose and sense of mattering. Pets have been effective in reducing blood pressure. They give an owner a reason to get better. Pet owners survive heart attacks in greater percentages than those without a pet at home, regardless of the human relationships surrounding the patient. Elderly Medicare pet owners were found to have less psychological distress and fewer doctor visits in a year than did non–pet owners, even if the individuals did not live alone. That may be why there are well over a hundred million cats and dogs in the United States.

In an institutional setting, animals can help individuals in ways humans may not be able to. They lessen fear and loneliness, thereby making adaptation to an institution easier. In addition, the ability to form an attachment to a pet generalizes to people. That is probably why many nursing homes permit animal visits. The sight of a cute animal lights up the faces of residents in a facility.

Resident pets used in therapy programs became catalysts for social interaction among both the patients and the staff. They helped socially isolated individuals to communicate with others and increase their self-esteem, so that these individuals participated more in group activities. Preliminary fears about the problems that might arise with a resident pet usually disappear after a few weeks. The animal provides affection and makes the unit it lives in more like home. Needless to say, it is important to select a pet with the right temperament.

There is no doubt that the loss of a pet brings on sadness and intensifies depression and anger. Nonetheless, the years of benefits outweigh the grief. A mourning period leads to renewal and teaches us that it is possible to heal and move on.

Religion teaches us the same thing. The expression "There are no atheists in foxholes" applies to many stressful situations, not just wartime. If you think that religion can be any kind of solace for you, there are various aspects to consider. First of all, no matter what your religion, you know that you can communicate to your Divine Being privately as well as within a place of worship. Talking directly to this Force gives you an outlet for your sadness, frustration, and anger. Praying in a congregational setting forces you to be presentable and to make even superficial contact with others. So, you can see that both ways of praying have their value.

You can turn to your religious leader for solace, but remember that even wise leaders are only human. As Rabbi Harold Kushner says in the first chapter of his book *When Bad Things Happen to Good People:* "I find it very hard to tell them that life is fair, that God gives people what they deserve and need. Time after time, I have seen families and even whole communities unite in prayer for the recovery of a sick person, only to have their hopes and prayers mocked. I have seen the wrong people get sick, the wrong people be hurt, the wrong people die young" (p. 7).

How then to start pulling out of your sadness? Comparing yourself to someone more unfortunate than you will not bring solace. The tragic hero Job asked many questions. He cried out for answers, but what he really needed was understanding and sympathy. Like most of us, he craved reassurance that he was still a good person. So, when you, the caregiver, ask questions of your religious leader, what you really need is not lessons in theology, but rather gentle support. You need strength and courage to deal with your difficulties, while understanding that your problems seem unfair. They're not your fault. No one can explain why you are burdened with them, any more than they can explain our existence.

You may be wondering why this had to happen to you. You may beg for help in whatever shape you can think of. Then, you may despair that relief is not in sight. Just keep in mind that the answer to your prayers can be "No." You must believe that the dark tunnel you are in does have a light at its end, and you will come out of it unexpectedly enriched and wiser.

You must guard against punishing yourself as a result of your loved one's illness. You are a victim along with your patient. If you see yourself as a bad person who has earned this calamity, you will drive away those who want to help. They will not know how to approach you, and so they will turn away. It's important not to let self-imposed loneliness make a bad situation worse.

On the other hand, you do not need to surround yourself with those who are more concerned with their own feelings and needs than with you. They try to help, but they make things worse because of their self-absorption. At least they come. So many others do not. It is difficult to see someone you care about suffering. As you have found out, many avoid the experience. That is why the caregiver of a person with dementia feels rejection and isolation added to helplessness.

The practical and emotional demands made on family members who care for dementia patients are well documented. This type of illness is one of the greatest tests of the durability of a family. A lot of researchers and clinicians have been interested in understanding the variations in adjustment of family members caring for older dementia patients. That adjustment depends on who the family member is and what support system is available.

Several studies have shown that sustained responsibility for dementia patients directly affects the emotional well-being of family members. Gregory Hinrichsen, Ph.D., of the Geriatric Psychiatry Service and Research Department of Hillside Hospital, a division of Long Island Jewish Medical Center in Glen Oaks, New York, has studied management strategies of family members of dementia caregivers. His study of 150 caregivers included spouses (36.1 percent), adult children (58.6 percent), and other related or non-related individuals (5.3 percent). Of the family members, 70.4 percent of the caregivers were female and 75 percent were married. Family members were, on average, 59.6 years of age. Forty percent of the patients were diagnosed with senile dementia of the Alzheimer's type, 17.4 percent with dementia secondary to cerebral vascular problems (such as stroke or multi-infarct dementia), 2.8 percent with dementia secondary to Parkinson's disease or alcohol abuse, and the remaining 39.8 percent were diagnosed with a variety of other forms of dementia.

Hinrichsen suggested that there were three main ways in which the caregivers dealt with patient problems: criticism, encouragement, and active management.

Criticism includes efforts to manage the patient by yelling, criticizing, or threatening. Caregivers who use this technique may say, for example, "I told my relative to stop doing things that caused worry because of what it did to me (or to other family members)," or "I asked my relative to explain why he/she was doing something, to draw his/her attention to his/her mistakes." I must confess that I myself tried coercion in my desperation and bewilderment. The result was a frightful scene on the front steps of the house with Newton clinging to the banister, sitting on a step, and kicking my helper and me away. The male helper and I were unable to pry his hand loose. The helper tried yanking him, and that only produced pain. Force was the wrong approach. A nineteen-year-old wiser than I handled a similar situation quite differently: When Newton refused to come into the house at another time, this young man just walked with him for only a few minutes.

He soon suggested that it was chilly, and Newton agreed and just turned around and came home.

We all react differently to different situations, but exasperation makes us do things we would normally consider unthinkable. One of the women in my support group sobbed as she related that, in utter frustration, she had hit her husband repeatedly with a hairbrush. She vowed never to do that again, only to end up hitting him with the same hairbrush a few days later. As heartwrenching as it was for her to place him in a nursing home, she felt that at least there, she would not beat him.

Encouragement means praising the patient or getting him/her to discuss feelings. Basically it involves giving emotional support. Caregivers using encouragement may say things like, "I made a point of praising him when he did what I considered appropriate," "I tried to engage my older relative in discussing his feelings and emotions," or "I showed special amounts of physical affection."

Hinrichsen found that managing the patient with criticism was associated with poorer adjustment of caregivers to their new roles, whereas the opposite was true with encouragement. The use of criticism was tied to a greater sense of burden, more psychiatric symptoms, and a greater desire on the part of the caregiver to institutionalize the patient.

Active management includes trying to safeguard, help, stimulate, and monitor the patient in order to modify the immediate environment or the daily routine. In Hinrichsen's study, greater active management was associated with a greater sense of burden and also a greater desire to institutionalize the patient. (The burden on family members and the availability of other people to assist the patient was also associated with physical health of the caregivers.) Those using active management might say things like, "I kept a close eye on what my older relative was doing so that I could head off any problems before they developed too far," "I tried to arrange my older relative's environment to safeguard her against causing problems, getting into trouble, or endangering herself," or "I tried to have my relative participate in as much of the ordinary family routine as possible."

Other studies concluded that different dementia management strategies did not have an impact on patient memory or behavior problems. This is a reminder that the disease you are dealing with is physical, not emotional. If you see your loved one's unusual behavior as being intentional, you will respond by trying to reason with him/her or by criticizing. However, you must realize that you really have no control over the situation. You can only control your reaction to it. Only when a friend of mine pointed out to me that Newton couldn't possibly want to wet himself intentionally did I realize, finally, that he was indeed not responsible for his actions. Our life together became much more pleasant after that. The coping strategies you use can work for or against you. The way you cope will influence your emotional state and vice versa.

The problems that come up when you are providing care to your loved one may overwhelm you. Your own survival might be at stake. That being the case, you should seek help at home or in a facility without guilt or embarrassment. Those of us who have personally experienced being a dementia caregiver will understand. None of us would criticize anyone else's coping techniques, whether they include at-home help or a nursing home. Devotion is personalized: You do what is right for you, never mind the know-it-alls.

Clinicians have observed that some family members can't delegate even the smallest amount of patient care, even when helpers are available. But there has to be a satisfactory balance between doing and not doing in dementia care. Such a balance won't be arrived at instantly. Through trial and error, using criticism (which will make matters worse), encouragement (which requires patience and perspective), or active management (which will increase your burden), you will develop the coping techniques that are most comfortable and successful for you. If coping with the burdens of caregiving is becoming a problem, definitely look into getting outside help. It has been documented that if the patient is receiving Medicaid, fewer needs had to be met only by the family, and more needs were met by the formal care network.

Some family members are more effective at dealing with dementia issues than are others. Of course, if you are the only one eligible to be the primary caregiver, you have little choice. You can, however, choose to develop techniques that will lessen stress. People who use avoidance techniques or wishful thinking to deal with their difficult situation have poorer emotional adjustment. On the other hand, people who accept the situation, focus on the positive, and reframe the problem have a better emotional adjustment. In other words, it all goes back to the old song about accentuating the positive and eliminating the negative This is not to suggest that dealing with a dementia patient is not overwhelming. The point is that you, the caregiver, will be less harried and share more warm feelings with your afflicted loved one if you choose to focus on whatever positive elements you can find. Handling the situation inappropriately will only increase stress in already stress-prone patients. It will also increase your own stress level and lead to anger and depression.

CHECKLIST

- ❑ Carefully select the few people you will want to call upon for emotional and physical support.
- ❑ Understand that ignorance makes friends and family members afraid of dealing with the person with dementia or with you, so reach out to them and be as patient as you can.
- ❑ Schedule daily activities that you can share with your loved one.
- ❑ Consider adopting an older pet who is already trained.
- ❑ Evaluate your attitude toward your religion and consider turning to your religious institution.

ADDITIONAL READING
ABOUT EMOTIONAL SUPPORT

Davis, Kathy Diamond. *Therapy Dogs.* New York: Howell Book House, 1992.
Hinrichsen, G. A., and G. Niederhe. "Dementia Management Strategies and Adjustment of Family Members of Older Patients." *Gerontologist* 34 (1994): 95–102.

Laland, Stephanie. *Animal Angels*. Berkeley, Calif.: Conari Press, 1998.

McElroy, Susan C. *Animals as Guides for the Soul*. New York: Ballantine Wellspring Books, 1998.

Oliver, Rose, and Frances A. Bock. *Coping with Alzheimer's: A Caregiver's Emotional Survival Guide*. New York: Dodd Mead and Co., 1987.

CHAPTER 5

Nursing Homes

Individuals with Alzheimer's/dementia make up the nursing home industry's fastest growing population. We all remember fondly stories of the "good old days" when the elderly were taken care of by their family, at home. The fact is, though, that in the past people usually didn't live long enough to burden their families with a dementing illness. Even if it was necessary to take care of elderly family members, "elderly" meant fifties or sixties. The caregivers were therefore much younger than today's children of ailing parents. Also, the elders had a shorter life span. That's why nursing homes are needed more nowadays.

Some nursing homes have received negative publicity that has given the entire industry a bad name. However, not all homes deserve criticism. Many facilities give good care and provide the best possible place for an impaired person. Continuing care retirement communities that offer assisted living can meet the needs of those in the beginning stages of dementia, but when someone needs constant care, being unable to bathe, eat, dress, and toilet him/herself, more individual assistance is necessary.

Just when should you place someone in a nursing home? When it is no longer possible to take care of your loved one at home or in an alternative living facility, or when the patient will for some reason be better off. Although you can monitor your loved one more carefully when he/she is at home, you can also be overwhelmed and ineffective. If the person with dementia becomes violent or uncontrollable even with medication, you must consider safety first. No matter what, the placement in a nursing home brings with it gut-wrenching guilt (warranted or not) and overwhelming sadness. If you needed support before, you need it more now. You know that you are doing the best thing possible for the patient and for you. If you became completely worn out, you wouldn't be of much help. You must stick by your decision, since you did not make it lightly.

Even if you do not see a need for a nursing home at the beginning, it is wise to plan ahead. There are shortages of beds for people with dementias. You will want to put your ward on the waiting list of a good facility well ahead of time. If you wait until it is necessary to transfer someone from a hospital stay, you may have to settle for whatever is available for a while, even if it doesn't offer the quality of care you want. Then you would have to transfer the patient and do double work as well as put your confused loved one through the stress of another adjustment.

Whom can you turn to in order to get help in making the right decision? Your closest relatives may be unable to listen. Your own children or siblings may have to tune out in order to deal with their own pain (or not face it at all). A nursing home eliminates your task of finding help at home. There will always be someone on staff in a facility. You may not like some of the workers, but they are not your responsibility. You just have to find the right nursing home!

Your first stop should be the public library. There are reference books that list nursing homes by area and categorize them in various ways. (*The Inside Guide to America's Nursing Homes,* in this chapter's suggested reading list, is a total resource all by itself.) The Internet is also a great supplier of information, at your fingertips. If you don't have Internet access, your library or friends may. The Alzheimer's Association is an excellent resource, too. The workers are knowledgeable and ready to give you useful information. In addition, they will put you in contact with a local support group and its social worker, who probably can give you a list of local nursing homes.

What research should you do before choosing a nursing home? At the very least, you want to make sure that the facility is licensed by the state in which it is located. There are various federal and state overseers you can contact to obtain information on different facilities. I looked under "Nursing Homes" in the yellow pages of my telephone book, and found four different organizations listed that give information about local nursing homes. Three out of the four charge no fee at all. The fourth charged for guiding someone through the process of choosing a facility, filling out forms, dealing with Medicaid, and so on. The fees depend on how much assistance you need. There are also a few dozen nursing homes listed in my directory. It will take you a long time to make all the phone calls, so you need to allow many days to pick out homes that you want to examine further. You should check out two to five nursing homes.

Whichever agencies supervise and evaluate nursing homes in your area should be doing the following:

▶ visiting the nursing home at least once a year

▶ having the visiting team include a nurse, a maintenance inspector, and a dietary expert conducting private interviews during which they visit and talk with individual residents and family members

▶ taking a number of days to thoroughly complete their inspection

▶ writing up a detailed evaluation, in the form of a survey report, which must be available for public review at all times

As you evaluate a nursing home, you want to pay close attention to the staff-to-patient ratio. In an ideal world, there would be one attendant for each resident. That's expensive. In reality, you want to see enough staff so that the patients are attended to promptly twenty-four hours a day. You don't want harried workers tending to your loved one.

Another thing you will want to know is whether this nursing home is owned by private individuals or by a corporation. A large corporation would be more likely to have the power to challenge regulations. These are the very regulations that protect the helpless.

Also find out whether the facility is run for profit or is part of a non-profit organization. The fees are higher for a profit-driven organization.

Ask for detailed fee schedules. The daily cost of nursing home care in the United States averages $115 per day, which adds up to $42,000 per year. Facilities in urban areas usually charge higher fees, due to the higher cost of labor. Individual nursing homes in the same locale do not necessarily charge the same fees. The quality of care in a nursing home is not related to its cost. Good care is less a result of dollars and cents than of compassion, expertise, hard work, attention to detail, and human dynamics.

Speaking of fees, keep in mind that, even though you may sign an admissions contract for someone else, you are not personally liable for the cost. If anyone tries to tell you otherwise, remind them that there is a law that protects you.

Find out whether or not there is a waiting list. There are people who have been able to place their loved one in a facility of their choice by paying the full fee for several months or a year. Then, when funds have been exhausted or the legal Medicaid requirements have been met, Medicaid took over the payments. An elder law attorney could figure out how the legal formula would work in each case. After receiving full payment for a while, the nursing home has been more willing to accept the Medicaid assignment. Those who don't have even a few months' payment must search to find a nursing home that will take Medicaid payments from the start of the patient's stay. In any case, fill out and file all applications for admission promptly.

You also should find out what the capacity of the nursing home is and how many patients are actually in residence. If there are lots of empty beds, you will want to know why. Does it mean that the facility earned a poor rating during the state's survey? On the other hand, if it is crowded, it may be understaffed, and that will result in poor care.

You will need a facility that allows you to visit freely and does not limit the visiting hours to a short period. It is always advisable to come at different times and on different days: You want to see that the patient is always cared for properly, not just when you are expected. You might want to be allowed to stay in the dining room during meals. Look at the menus—are there alternatives to the meals available? Does the food look appetizing? If your patient has dietary restrictions, make sure they are taken care of. Outside the dining room, can a resident keep a glass of water by his bedside? If not, will someone bring water during the night?

Once you have narrowed down the possible choices, visit each facility yourself. Make an appointment to speak to the director. To whom can you communicate complaints or praise? Are suggestions welcome? Ask for the facility's most recent inspection survey. If it shows violations, ask how they have been remedied. While you're there, walk around, look, listen, and smell. Urine is practically odorless unless it is left for hours, in which case it develops an ammonia smell. Ask how the staff monitors the need for diaper changes of incontinent patients. Other odors, like those of strong cleaning products, are also undesirable. All cleaning products should be locked away. If there is carpeting in the resident areas, find out how toilet accidents are handled. Carpeting can retain odors and germs for a long time.

Ask to visit at least two patient quarters. Check for cleanliness in both the bedroom and the bathroom. Verify that bed linens and towels are changed daily. In the bathroom, turn on the water to check the water pressure and temperature, as well as ease of operation of the faucets. Be aware of the temperature in the room. If it is too cold or too hot, find out why and ask about individual thermostats. Excessive heat dries out the skin and nasal passages, leading to rashes and nosebleeds. Find out how often routine showers and baths are given. Take a look at the bathing facilities: Is the equipment adequate and safe?

When you visit a nursing home, you can sense whether or not the staff cares. A high employee turnover rate affects the consistency of care, and is a tip-off to dissatisfied workers. No employees should be yelling or using abusive language. In addition, their speech should be easily understood. Heavy foreign accents are hard for anyone to understand, but even harder to comprehend and more frustrating for someone with dementia. The workers should be neat and clean. If they are union members, ask who takes over in case of a strike. Those in contact with the residents should be sensitive to their needs and should not, for example, wear heavy perfume or have long nails that can scratch fragile skin.

You will most likely see a lineup of residents seated in their wheelchairs near the elevator. They are scrubbed clean. Are they tied down? Only extreme cases should be, if a medical condition warrants restraint. The halls should be clean and well lit, with handrails for support. Check the rails to see that they are secure. There should be no accessible or frayed electric wires. Corridors should be wide enough for wheelchairs to roll through without difficulty.

Since you are placing a demented patient, look for special accommodations such as areas that are safe for a resident to wander in. A circular corridor may be bothersome to a visitor, but the fact that it doesn't have a dead end enables a dementia/Alzheimer's patient to wander about safely. A wander-guard alarm system, something like an invisible fence, protects an unpredictable resident from excessive wandering. However, that might mean that the resident is never allowed to step outside.

Are the walls decorated with appropriate topics referring to current happenings? You want your needy loved one to be as stimulated as possible within the limitations imposed by the disease. Even a person with dementia needs physical stimulation. So you want to know whether there is a physical therapist available, and how often therapy is provided. Good nursing homes pride themselves in organized activities that bring some variety to the day-to-day lives of the residents. The staff brings individuals to the group area rather than leaving them in their rooms to stare at the four walls. Even if the patient doesn't fully understand or participate, the change will do him/her good. Music, especially, has special charms. You would be amazed to hear someone otherwise quite "out of it" sing along at a song fest!

Test the furniture you see to make sure it is in good working condition. The walls and furniture do not have to be bland. I've seen colorful Formica dressers as well as wood-like beds and desks (which served more for storing underwear than for writing on) that made you feel as though the living quarters were not overly institutional. The more home-like the environment is, the less depressing it will be for you and the resident.

At the time of admission, bring along a list of the medication your loved one is on. Also bring some basic clothes and label them, but do not bring fine-quality clothing. Your relation will end up being dressed in outfits you have never seen before. It is hopeless to try to figure out what happened to the clothes you brought. You have to be grateful that he/she is being kept clean and warm. It might be possible for you to bring home the laundry. That would give you a little more control over the wardrobe, but you still will have surprises. It may not be the carelessness of the staff that results in missing or exchanged clothing: it is typical for Alzheimer's residents to take the belongings of others.

Most of the time, the advice given to family members of newly admitted patients with dementia is hard to follow. They are told not to visit for the first few days. That is to enable the patient to get adjusted to the new environment. It can be torture for you, though. If you can't handle it, talk to the home's social worker and work out a more satisfactory arrangement. What could happen if you do come for a visit at the beginning of the stay? Your loved one may implore you to be taken home. You know that isn't feasible. You may have to slip away when you leave. It seems sneaky, but it's survival. You can't explain or reason with that person—that's why you had to place him/her in the nursing home to begin with! Then, when the day comes that the person you love, even in this condition, doesn't even look up when you arrive, there's another stab of pain.

Once you start visiting on a regular basis, it's a good idea to plan what you are going to try to talk about. Tell the patient what's happening in the family and the old neighborhood. Share problems as well as happy events. Even people in an altered mental state are not too fragile to deal with sadness and death. Besides, protecting them may make them feel left out, and they have a right to know, even if that knowledge disappears almost instantly. Even if you get no feedback, it will do you good to talk about what is on your mind. Occasionally include your patient's roommate(s) in your conversations. This encourages relationships, as limited as they might be, and it shows your genuine interest in the present environment. If you think it's appropriate, bring things to read aloud or a very basic game to play. Help decorate the room with photos and plants.

When your loved one expresses feelings of distress, empathize. Denying the existence of these feelings will not help you or the patient. At times, this support has nothing to do with reality: it may not be true that someone stole something, but true or not, the event in the patient's mind is upsetting, and he/she needs soothing. Don't feel your relative is angry at you specifically. A sympathetic ear will go a long way. However, should the complaint be legitimate, it is up to you, the capable one, to assess situations surrounding the one you care about. If you feel that the problem warrants a change of room, insist on a modification of the situation. You are the advocate, and need not be shy. At the same time, you should avoid making an issue of relatively minor details because you will not be listened to when you need to make a valid complaint.

Should the resident be too demented to respond in any way, you can still talk and touch. You can also meet a family member or close friend there and catch up on old times. Your loved one may be past understanding, but he/she is not past feeling. It will alleviate your sense of helplessness to reach out in some way, as long as you don't expect the impossible. Go for a walk with your loved one, pushing him/her in a wheelchair if need be. Even a visit to the lobby will be a change of scene beneficial to both of you.

Another way you can feel useful is to share some of your skills and talents with others. If you play a musical instrument, sing, or can do artwork, you might lead other patients more capable than yours in a pleasant activity. You can also visit a lonely resident whose disabilities are physical. That way, your visits benefit residents who are more aware of their surroundings, and thoughtful acts replenish your soul. Ask one of the social workers to guide you toward a needy patient.

The office of social services has trained social workers who will do their best to be supportive and help you out. They often coordinate the admission process and provide counseling to residents and families on coping with the emotional stress of illness. They help make decisions regarding continuity of care and sometimes conduct support groups for residents and families. However, they often have a heavy caseload that doesn't leave too much time for chats other than in emergency situations. In addition, they are required to discuss money matters with family members, and that eats up more of their time.

Should Alzheimer patients be intermingled with other types of residents, or in a section with only demented patients? There are two schools of thought, which each have pros and cons. If demented residents are integrated with the general population, they will get more intellectual stimulation, but the other patients might be upset by them. The staff might be impatient with people who cannot communicate properly. On the other hand, if these residents are in their own section, they will not stand out as misfits and their aides will not be as likely to be annoyed at their behavior. However, they will be surrounded by people with advanced dementia, who might disturb them and certainly won't stimulate them.

Only you can decide which way makes you less uncomfortable. If you don't have a choice, it's that much less that you will have to lose sleep over. In any case, though, make sure that the facility does currently care for people with dementia. If not, this place is not the right choice.

There are a few rare places in which Alzheimer's patients have an environment tailor-made for them: in certain assisted living facilities, the residents have greater freedom, are encouraged to make choices, and are surrounded by specially trained staff. They receive appropriate stimuli and handling. Needless to say, such a setting is only appropriate as long as the resident is ambulatory. One such facility, in California, places "think boxes" all around to help patients exercise the healthy parts of their minds. "Memory boxes" are outside their rooms to help them identify their quarters and to give a synopsis of their accomplishments and highlight their life's events.

For those who like to roam (a persistent problem when you have the patient at home), there are "wandering paths" with gardens and beautiful views. The patients can't open the attractive gate in the fence that surrounds the grounds. The staff keeps a watchful eye on the roamers, and they come back on their own or are guided back. For the inevitable hostile moods, there is a bean wheel. It hangs on the wall, easily available to staff members. This transparent circle contains brightly colored beans. When someone spins the wheel, the falling beans create bright images that attract attention, and the resident who is behaving inappropriately is distracted long enough to stop his/her negative behavior. There are also phones that only play music and serve as audio distractions. (Maybe you would like to incorporate some of these gimmicks into your own home before a transfer to a nursing home becomes necessary.)

Although such residences are a treat to visit, you can't count on finding one in your area. So you must do your homework and find the best facility you can in this less-than-perfect world you are dealing with. With proper guidance and support, you will be able to handle the situations as they present themselves. Unfortunately, upsetting situations will crop up in any facility you have chosen. Watch for drug overdoses or drug interaction problems. If you see a sudden change in appearance or behavior, question what's behind it. Your loved one is helpless. You don't have the control you had at home, but you can certainly question whatever seems puzzling. If an answer doesn't satisfy you, go to the person at the next higher level. It is, unfortunately, easy to overmedicate or mismedicate someone who is unable to express feelings and sensations. It is also more convenient to have a patient safely in a wheelchair than walking around and getting into mischief, bothering the other residents as well as the staff. Be alert and in touch enough to evaluate what you see.

Should you tip the employees? Some facilities have firm policies against it; some are more lenient. You can always bring some goodies to eat, or a thoughtful gift if you can't or don't want to give money. Listen to your sixth sense on this. If a patient is pleasant and easy to care for, the staff will want to be around him/her more than if the patient is mean or obnoxious. That also will influence your decision about tipping. Keep in mind that a resident cannot be dismissed from a nursing home because of personality conflicts. Only health or safety concerns give the nursing home the right to discharge someone.

How are you going to pay for all this? Medicare doesn't cover nursing home care that is not a medical necessity. Your loved one needs maintenance care. Is he/she eligible for Veterans Administration benefits? Will you need Medicaid? At what point? Is there a long-term-care policy or other coverage that applies? These things are discussed in detail in chapter 6.

In the nursing home, there is often one doctor on the floor, and outside doctors are not allowed to come in. If that is the case, check with the floor doctor to see what his program of care is, including medications and treatments. If your loved one's physician is allowed to follow the patient in the nursing home and is willing to do so, that's fine. However, if you must now find a new doctor, look for one who is a certified geriatrician and who has admitting privileges in one of the hospitals the nursing home deals with. If a specific medical problem develops, the patient will have to be transferred to a nearby hospital, where there is a further supply of physicians. The nursing home bed is reserved for a limited time and under a variety of circumstances—ask the nursing home for specifics.

There have been unscrupulous directors of nursing homes who have taken advantage of a patient's hospital stay to force the patient out of the home; saying that the bed is no longer available, the director will push out an undesirable resident rather than find another bed within a short time. What makes a patient "undesir-able"? One of the primary reasons for expelling a resident is the fact that he/she is on Medicaid. In many states, there are clear laws against such practices. Look in the yellow pages for an agency that supports relatives or friends of the institutionalized aged. You can also contact the National Citizens' Coalition for Nursing Home Reform in Washington, D.C. These organizations will tell you what laws you can turn to for help.

When your loved one does have to be temporarily transferred to a hospital for a medical procedure, you will want to know that the hospital is a good one. How can you know how good the hos-pital is? In this case also, the cost of care is not a reliable indicator of quality. You want to see that the hospital has accreditation from the federal Joint Commission on Accreditation of Healthcare Orga-nizations (JCAHO). That means that the hospital meets certain minimal standards. The Joint Commission is an independent, non-profit organization that conducts a quality assessment of most hospitals every three years. Although this process is voluntary, about 80 percent of U.S. hospitals participate.

There are different levels of accreditation: Most hospitals receive simple accreditation, and only a few receive accreditation with commendation, conditional accreditation, or no accreditation. If a hospital has received conditional accreditation, it has six months to correct the deficiencies found in the quality assess-ment. You are entitled to know when the commission last surveyed the hospital, and when the next survey will occur. To check, ask to speak to someone in the quality management department. If need be, you can call the JCAHO service center at (708) 916-5800. They will also send you a detailed report on a facility for a fee. This report covers nursing care, infection control, patient rights, and safety. Another sign of quality in a hospital is a large number of board-certified physicians on its staff.

Once you have assured yourself that the hospital is adequate, you must deal with the decisions involved in treating the specific ailment for which your loved one is being hospitalized. Before you give permission for any procedure to be done, you should ask several questions, such as:

— What is the purpose of the procedure?
— What are the side effects?
— What kind of recuperation is required?
— What will be the improvement?
— How does this improvement compare to the risks?

As you ask such questions, keep in mind that the person for whom you are making decisions is suffering from an irreversible, deteriorating disease. Also keep in mind what this individual's general physical health is.

When your loved one enters the hospital, verify that all necessary legalities are on file. If there is a DNR (do not resuscitate) order, be sure the medical staff is aware of it. Make sure there are copies of a living will and a health care proxy in the hands of all those who have the power to make decisions. You want to be the one to make the ultimate decisions, following what you knew were the wishes of your once-coherent loved one.

Whether your loved one is temporarily in a hospital or more permanently in a nursing home, you are going to be alone. You will no longer have the hourly struggles, but neither will you have a purpose to your days. You must now give some structure to your life. A support group would give you some structure. This is also a good time to join an exercise class because physical exertion cleanses the mind. Begin a creative project. It will give you a needed escape from reality. Your ordeal is not over. You will face many empty hours. Reach out, do what you think you want to do. You can always change your mind.

You have lost control over so much, but you can still arrange your own activities. Renew yourself with whatever gives you satisfaction. You deserve some of the good things in life, and now is the time to begin reintroducing yourself to them.

CHECKLIST

❑ Research possible nursing homes and regulatory agencies (see the suggested reading list).

❑ Make appointments to visit each nursing home you are considering, and come equipped with your own personal checklist and questions.

❑ Discuss financial details with the appropriate staff.

❑ Learn the rules and regulations of each facility and make sure that you can live with them.

❑ Check for safety features, look for decorations that remind patients of dates and holidays, and sit in on a group activity.

❑ Walk through the hallways, look into empty rooms and trust your gut instinct.

❑ Label the clothes and personal possessions that you intend to bring to the home.

❑ Find ways to deal with your visits and don't hesitate to correct situations you see as harmful to your loved one's well-being.

❑ Seek out a support system.

❑ Start structuring your day to include some creative activity.

ADDITIONAL READING ABOUT NURSING HOMES

Bua, Robert N. *The Inside Guide to America's Nursing Homes (Rankings and Ratings for Every Nursing Home in the U.S.)*. New York: Warner Books, 1998–99.

Kranz, Marian R. *The Nursing Home Choice: How to Choose the Ideal Nursing Home*. Brookline Village, Mass.: Branden Publishing, 1998.

CHAPTER 6

Finances

You have heard the dreaded diagnosis. What should you do to protect your assets and keep them from being completely depleted? Ideally, one should not wait for a crisis to do advance planning. At this point, it's crucial not to wait any longer. Go to an elder law attorney for a consultation.

What elder law is best known for today is dealing with this question: If I (or someone close to me) become sick and require long-term care, how am I going to be able to afford that care in my area? Elder law is the legal specialty that deals with the specific concerns of senior citizens. It is a developing area of law, and many people don't know that it exists. As our population ages, more and more people will need this specialized advice.

Even if you have few assets, it is well worth the time and money to see a professional about what your options are. If the patient is already on Medicaid, you should contact Medicaid to find out what your loved one will be entitled to. The more informed you are, the more prepared you will be to make the decisions that will present themselves throughout an illness.

How do you go about choosing an elder law attorney? Choose one that specializes in that field. Seek recommendations from other professionals, such as geriatric care managers like caseworkers in the hospital, social workers, or gerontologists. Avoid someone who just advertises that he/she does elder law. Steven H. Stern, of Davidow, Davidow, Siegel and Stern, LLP, in Islandia, N.Y., suggested the following questions you can ask a lawyer in this field you're thinking of hiring:

— What percentage of your practice is devoted to elder law? How many elder law–related cases are new to your office every month, on the average?
— What are some of the issues your elder law cases involve?
— Aside from elder law cases, what percentage of your clients are senior citizens? (You want to make sure that this attorney knows how to deal with senior citizens on a variety of levels. Older people require compassion and understanding of their needs, besides needing financial knowledge. You will need a sympathetic ear as well as a knowledgeable guide.)
— Are you a member of the National Academy of Elder Law Attorneys?
— Are you an active member of your local and state bar association's elder law committee or section?
— Have you published articles or spoken to groups on this topic?

Some other questions might be:

— Is your office handicapped accessible?
— Is the seating appropriate for seniors, that is, is it easy to get in and out of?
— How long a wait can I expect, both in the waiting room and to have papers finalized?

If someone is diagnosed with dementia early on, he/she still has the capacity to function. Someone who has just been diagnosed still knows who he/she is and can still participate in planning for the future. At the time of diagnosis there is a window of opportunity when it is still possible for the patient to manage financial affairs. It's important to take advantage of this remaining time. You, the caregiver, must explain this situation to your patient. Too often too much time is allowed to pass before planning begins, and people are unprepared for the inevitable financial burdens that arise.

Planning ahead is an opportunity to take control of the situation. If someone has a stroke, its effects are catastrophic—you don't have the choice of making any arrangements after the fact.

However, in the case of dementia, the patient is still the same person he/she was an hour before going to the doctor's office. Point out to your loved one that knowing something needs to be done before the disease progresses gives him/her an opportunity to be remembered for the steps he/she takes now, while he/she is still lucid and rational enough to accomplish the necessary goals. You should use all the influence you have to make sure that you both follow through on plans because ultimately, the burden will be on you.

What kinds of financial concerns should be addressed at this point? Decisions need to be made about paying the bills and taxes, managing investments, keeping up insurance, and maintaining the patient's home. Future patient care has to be anticipated, too. Somebody must have the authority to handle these matters.

People with a frightening diagnosis are probably also concerned that medical decisions be made according to their wishes if they become unable to communicate. Besides these immediate concerns, it is now necessary to think about estate planning, probate and inheritance taxes, and disabled children or grandchildren.

To get the ball rolling, the first order of business is to give a spouse or other trusted individual a power of attorney. If there is no such document available when someone is unable to make financial transactions, someone will need to start a guardianship proceeding. That is time-consuming and frustrating. It also means the decision is made by a judge first, rather than by family members. These decisions may not be what the once-competent patient would have wanted. A trip to the courthouse also opens the door for family squabbles. It is therefore in everyone's best interest to resolve all possible legal and financial matters when the patient is able. If guardianship is acquired, or a power of attorney is signed, it is possible for the designated person to make financial moves on behalf of the incapacitated person. That could include the necessary transfers to qualify for Medicaid.

Since financing long-term care is the greatest concern, you must explore the different options to fund this great expense.

Your first option is to pay for it yourself. That will usually involve a progression from day care to an adult home to a nursing home. You should have a discussion with your elder law attorney about admission requirements and contracts. This is an intimidating time for the caregiver, since you want the best you can get for your loved one, but you don't want to be taken advantage of. It helps to be aware of some myths about care. It isn't true that you have to take the first bed available within a certain mile radius, or that you have to pay for a certain number of months up front in order to be admitted, or that if you are discharged back to a hospital from a nursing home, you are going to lose your bed (see chapter 5 on nursing homes).

It is a violation of federal law to insist that a child assume personal liability for payment of a parent's bill. However, a spouse can be held liable, even if there has been a prenuptial agreement and funds have been kept separate. It is also a violation of federal law for someone to have you waive your rights to Medicare or Medicaid. If a nursing home should insist on any of these provisions, call a good elder law attorney who can serve as your advocate. A call to the nursing home from such an attorney, pointing out that the home is in violation of federal and state nursing home regulations, will go a long way.

Just because you start as a private paying patient does not mean that you have to continue paying until you have spent all of your money. Your patient can become eligible for Medicaid before either of you becomes destitute. The patient can also switch from private funding to Medicaid once he/she has entered the nursing home. There are two ways of looking at the situation. One view is: "My loved one's savings were put away for a rainy day, and therefore should be used toward the cost of daily care." Another view is: "Wouldn't it be devastating to spend an entire life's savings and then have to go on Medicaid anyway?" Many consider it better to go on Medicaid early on, thus protecting assets for the patient and others, rather than allowing all the accumulated funds to disappear and then have to count on Medicaid after all. Besides money, emotions are important, too: people who are totally dependent on the government feel they've lost control since they can't take financial action on their own.

Caregivers may feel like thieves, ripping off the system. They may feel that they have to do Medicaid planning in secrecy and hide assets. Or they may feel it is up to them to be heroes and preserve a lifetime of savings for the loved one. They also can't help but think of their own inheritance. How can one reconcile these feelings? First, it is important to remember that there are rules and regulations that allow us to protect assets without committing fraud. Nursing home costs are exorbitant, and so it doesn't take long to spend the savings from a lifetime of hard work. Many feel there is no way they could have planned responsibly for this contingency, especially since there was no good long-term-care insurance available as recently as ten years ago. Even nowadays, such insurance is costly and hard to qualify for.

Can you consider Medicare a reliable source of payment for nursing home care? Unfortunately, no. The Alzheimer's/dementia patient is not going to benefit much from Medicare, whose typical recipient has suffered a catastrophic illness such as a stroke or a broken hip and been taken to a hospital. After a hospital stay, such a patient then needs to go into a skilled nursing facility. Once a patient needs this level of skilled nursing care, Medicare will cover the stay in an extended-care facility. The skilled care consists of rehabilitative and therapeutic assistance, such as physical, speech, and occupational therapy. This assistance will enable the patient to recover, and then be sent home.

Since typical Alzheimer's/dementia patients are able to get along on their own for a while, they only need assistance when difficulties increase. Then that need for assistance grows until it is no longer possible for such patients to stay home (unless the home is set up like a mini–nursing home). These people might then need nursing home care, but they will not be coming from a hospital stay. Therefore Medicare will pay for nothing. As for signing up for long-term-care insurance, it is no longer an option after the diagnosis.

That leaves Medicaid, which is a joint federal and state program. It is the principal public method for funding nursing home care, paying for 45 percent of all nursing home costs in the United States. It comprises almost 90 percent of government expenditures for such care. It is the payer of last resort.

There are a number of reasons to engage in Medicaid planning for the benefit of someone diagnosed with Alzheimer's. This planning goes above and beyond merely preserving someone's inheritance. Medicaid pays room and board in a nursing home, but doesn't pay for other expenses. An institutionalized individual gets only a small resource allowance for personal needs from Medicaid. This allowance is a very small portion of his/her monthly income. In some states, the allowance is $30.00. Weekly visits to the nursing home hairdresser, clothing, and so forth will more than deplete that allotment. What if additional care is needed within the nursing home? Private care is not covered by Medicaid. Neither are some other personal needs. Not to be able to pay for such "extras" is demoralizing. Any amount of money a recipient gets above the personal needs allowance is the "net available monthly income" that is payable to the nursing home.

Because Medicaid is a program designed to provide medical assistance to the needy, there are several financial restrictions to deal with: applicants can only be eligible if they have minimal income and assets that must be available to be counted toward eligibility requirements. Social Security and pension benefits are included. In the case of a married couple, both spouses' gross monthly income counts. The amount and types of assets acceptable vary among the states. Some assets do not count toward Medicaid eligibility. However, any transfer of assets during the last three years (the "lookback period") renders a Medicaid applicant ineligible.

Even if you have no intention of filing a Medicaid application at this time, you should write to your local Medicaid eligibility program's assessment unit to request an assessment of the total value of your combined countable resources. Contact the Federal Department of Health and Human Services for details. Remember that, for Medicare assistance, you should go to your nearest Social Security office, and for Medicaid assistance, you should contact your state or local welfare office. There are often times when one program can be used in conjunction with the other. If you have trouble locating the appropriate organization, your local senior center may be able to give you guidance in this matter.

It is only when the resources of an applicant and the applicant's spouse are reduced to allowable levels that he/she can obtain Medicaid coverage. These levels are determined by individual states. Also, applicants must ask for all the benefits to which they are entitled and any private medical payments they receive to be assigned to the Medicaid agency.

A routine strategy used to make someone eligible for Medicaid is to simply transfer assets to another person, preferably to a spouse. Federal tax law permits unlimited transfers between spouses and allows gifts of up to $10,000 to as many people as one wants without having to file any forms. However, many people don't want to transfer their assets to someone else because they don't want to lose control, or would suffer adverse tax consequences (such as loss of tax exemptions for real estate), or because they fear family problems such as divorce or bankruptcy. So transferring assets outright may not be the best choice, especially with the three-year waiting period.

Another option is the use of special deeds and trusts. Special trusts used in a Medicaid context can be very sophisticated and at times complicated to use. It is important to keep in mind that only trusts that are irrevocable in nature can move you toward qualifying for Medicaid. Although revocable trusts are useful to manage assets upon incapacity and to avoid probate, they will do nothing to protect assets from the cost of long-term care. There is huge variation from state to state in the possible configuration of trusts, so these options must be discussed thoroughly with a competent and well-informed professional in your area.

Although the general rule says that a period of ineligibility is imposed on "uncompensated transfers of assets," there is an exception that allows a transfer between spouses without the imposition of a penalty period. That is a federal law that provides that an "institutional spouse" may transfer assets to a "community spouse" without penalty. A "community spouse" is the spouse of someone in an institution (such as a nursing home), and the "institutional spouse" is the person in a facility. The community spouse is guaranteed some level of self-sufficiency by keeping an allowable income and certain resources for his/her use.

One of these resources is the family home. It is possible to shelter funds by paying off the mortgage and making major repairs or alterations. Household goods and personal effects also do not count toward the total assets evaluated for Medicaid eligibility. Prepaying real estate taxes and funeral arrangements, as well as homeowner's insurance and utilities before the date of the Medicaid application is also allowed. An annuity is another possibility, but a commercial annuity has a large downside since the principal amount used to purchase it goes to the financial institution. To avoid that, one can enter into a private annuity agreement with family members. One should also consider a self-canceling installment note (SCIN) that may have more beneficial tax consequences than a private annuity.

Under federal law, the community spouse may not only hold on to certain income and resources, but in some states may also exercise "a right of spousal refusal." That means that a spouse can refuse to contribute any assets in his/her name toward the cost of the other spouse's care. The applicable laws that deal with this issue, like the social service law in some states, specify that Medicaid must be provided to the institutionalized spouse if the community spouse fails or refuses to contribute toward the institutionalized spouse's cost of care. However, if a spouse refuses support, the Medicaid eligibility program may refer the matter to court for a review of the spouse's actual ability to pay. The ramifications of such actions need to be studied and evaluated.

There are other transfers that may be made without subjecting the Medicaid applicant to a period of ineligibility. An applicant may transfer a house without penalty to a disabled child, to one who is under twenty-one, to a sibling who has some equity in the home and lived there for at least a year, or to a child of anyone who lived with the parent and took care of him/her for at least two years. It is also possible to transfer assets to someone else for the sole benefit of a spouse. Such a trust would be managed by a trustee for the benefit of the spouse. One can also transfer funds to or from a disabled child.

You may have heard about criminal penalties for transferring assets to qualify for Medicaid. The laws concerning this issue have vague elements that have been challenged in court and may or may not apply to your situation. Again, a competent elder law attorney can guide you. What about the law making it a crime for a paid advisor to "knowingly and willfully counsel or assist" someone to dispose of assets for the purpose of obtaining state-funded medical assistance? It, too, is subject to various interpretations because the language of the statute is ambiguous when determining whether or not a crime has been committed. There is also the possibility that that law infringes upon the First Amendment right to free speech by prohibiting a legal or financial advisor from counseling a client about activities that are legal. As you can see, there are more rules and interpretations than a layperson can handle alone.

Once Medicaid has approved an institutionalized spouse, the income from both spouses is used to determine applicable personal allowances and liabilities. If income is paid only in the name of the institutionalized spouse, that income is only available to that spouse. If it is payable to both spouses, one half of the income is considered to be available to each of them. If a trust distributes income, the trust agreement controls which income is attributable to each spouse. Your local library should have the latest charts available on Medicaid eligibility standards in each state for nursing homes.

If the patient is an eligible veteran, it is possible that the Veterans Administration might cover most of the costs of a nursing home stay, if not all the costs. All honorable and general discharge veterans are eligible for care, whether they served in a war or not. The patient would have to reside in a Veterans Administration facility, and be treated at a VA hospital. The requirement for eligibility is that the attending physician in a VA hospital must make the recommendation for transfer to a nursing home. If such facilities are near your home, contact the Veterans Administration without delay so that you can put your loved one's name on a waiting list and have a bed available when the time comes. Although the facilities may not be luxurious, the care is generally quite adequate.

Let's suppose that the one you are caring for has no spouse, and has little in the way of assets, except for his/her primary residence. As a general rule, a state must recover costs incurred from nursing home residency of a Medicaid patient who was fifty-five years old or older when benefits were received. Generally, the costs are recovered from the patient's estate, and states have the option of seeking recovery from any other assets in which the individual had any legal title or interest at the time of death. So once the primary residence is sold, some of the proceeds of that sale will have to go to repay Medicaid. Other assets, such as bank accounts, can also be tapped for reimbursement. Although states have the option of seeking recovery from property held through "joint tenancy," "tenancy in common," "life estate," "living trust," or other forms of ownership, many states have not exercised this option.

So what about planning for your own eventual long-term-care needs? Perhaps the best solution is long-term-care insurance, if you can get it. Such insurance provides for at-home or nursing home care for a specific amount of time and at a specific rate of coverage. The greater the coverage, the higher the premiums. Most policies are rather expensive. If you can't qualify for a policy or can't afford one, you have to explore other options, including Medicaid and its accompanying transfers of assets. Whether these transfers are in the form of a life estate or an irrevocable trust, it is important to study tax and legal consequences before proceeding.

In summary, what should you do the day your loved one is diagnosed? See to it that a power of attorney, health care proxy, and living will are drawn up right away. Then, find out what kind of care your insurance will cover. Check into your spouse's eligibility for Medicare, Medicaid, or other benefits such as veteran's benefits that may be used to cover costs. Most of all, look into the options suggested by a knowledgeable, competent elder law attorney.

What happens if these preparations aren't made? There will be guardianship or conservatorship proceedings, which involve going to court to have a loved one declared incompetent or incapacitated. You don't want to have to go to court: It's costly and time-consuming, and you have to live by a court order. You no longer have the flexibility to do things as you see fit, because you have to ask a judge for permission before you act. You have to account to the court every year. Also, if there is any family infighting about who should be the guardian, the court might appoint someone who is not a family member. Then it's the luck of the draw.

Since some people with dementing illnesses such as Alzheimer's can become defensive and accusatory, they might not want to sign any document perceived as loss of control. So, it falls upon you, the caregiver, to point out all the positives and the reasons why you must have a power of attorney. With that in hand, you can proceed to protect both your loved one and yourself. You want to start taking these important steps at a point when you and the patient are still able to, and before other family members become involved. It is by planning ahead that you will maintain control: you will continue to be able to make decisions about your finances even though you will be unable to control the inevitable progress of the disease. Doing nothing is losing control. You must hold the reins. That is the only way you can help yourself and thus help your loved one.

CHECKLIST

☐ Draw up a power of attorney, health care proxy, and living will. Don't wait.

☐ Ask around to find a competent elder law attorney.

☐ Interview as many attorneys as necessary to find one that suits you. Ask appropriate questions (see the first two pages of this chapter).

☐ Look for books in the library that will enable you to be more informed.

☐ Remember that you are doing nothing illegal by applying for Medicaid.

ADDITIONAL READING ABOUT FINANCES

Barnett, Terry James. *Living Wills and More: Everything You Need to Ensure That All Your Medical Wishes Are Followed.* New York: John Wiley and Sons, 1993.

Bove, Alexander A. *The Medicaid Planning Handbook: A Guide to Protecting Your Family's Assets from Catastrophic Nursing Home Costs.* New York: Little, Brown and Company, 1996.

Gordon, Harley, and Jane Daniel. *How to Protect Your Life Savings from Catastrophic Illness and Nursing Homes.* Boston: Financial Planning Institute, 1990.

Hynes, Margaret N. *Who Cares for Poor People? Physicians, Medicaid, and Marginality.* Florence, Ky.: Garland, 1998.

Williams, Phil. *The Living Will and the Durable Power of Attorney for Health Care Book: With Forms.* Oak Park, Ill.: Gaines, 1991.

CHAPTER 7

The Last
Chapter in
Your Patient's Life

No matter how much death is anticipated, when it actually comes, it's a shock. In preparing for the inevitable, there are major decisions to be made. If you have found your family supportive during your ordeal and you would like their input, by all means, talk to them about how to handle your loved one's death. But it is your decision, and no one really can do it for you, just as they couldn't lift that burden of caregiving off your shoulders. Remember also that you are bound to displease someone. If you and your patient have talked about death and know what he/she really wants, go to it and know you're following a loved one's final wishes. If someone else objects, you can quietly say, "That was what the deceased wanted."

Over the years, I was able to get Newton's input on certain details, even though he never wanted to talk about death. I would preface my question with what I wanted for myself, and then ask him what he would want. We could never have any long discussion on the subject, and so I ended up still getting information about details during lucid moments of his final illness.

By the way, during the times when the patient's mind still seems clear, bring up old grudges as well as sweet moments from the past. Clearing the air will ease your mourning and healing period down the road.

If you and the patient are both comfortable having him/her die at home, you should do some preparatory work. Talk it over. Ask a doctor to give a referral to home hospice care ahead of time. That will spare you great uncertainty, a house filled with police and EMS workers, and long waits for the coroner's office to approve the removal of the body. The hospice nurses are incredibly gentle and knowledgeable. They share their knowledge and minister to the sick with no hesitation.

Hospice nurses give medical care and pain management. They address the emotional, social, and spiritual needs of the patient and the family. They support the caregiver. They know how to handle grief. We don't know what to expect—what each change or symptom means—but they do. Their reassurance is precious.

They do a lot more than reassure: if your doctor can certify that the patient is terminal, the hospice nurses will come to your home and tend to all the needs of the patient. What a relief! I'm sorry that I didn't plan for that. I ended up being very much on my own at the hardest of times. The aide I had hired walked out. Had it not been for some dear friends, I don't know how I would have managed, since it was the weekend and Newton's doctors were not available. The dial-a-doctor I found in the yellow pages was out of town. When, at last, he was back, and Newton was comatose but still breathing, that doctor made the referral to the local hospice.

It was the hospice nurse who, at 1:00 A.M., asked to hear the sound of Newton's breathing on the phone. She reassured me that it was not unusual. (His death rattle had lasted for almost two days.) She is the one I called when he was no longer breathing. She guided me with wisdom and compassion. Had a hospice nurse started to care for Newton earlier, she would have been empowered to sign the death certificate, thus sparing me long delays before the coroner gave approval for the removal of the body. Instead, I had to call 911 and end up hosting two shifts of police because the coroner was unavailable for several hours. I was able to convince the EMS team members who pronounced the death (at the time they came, not at the time it happened) not to send the body to a hospital by ambulance. When that happens, a hospital staff member pronounces the patient "dead on arrival," and you get ambulance and hospital bills.

Most hospice care in the United States is paid for by Medicare if services are provided at home. To qualify for this benefit, beneficiaries must be covered by Medicare Part A and have a doctor certify that they have less than six months to live.

The hospice benefit covers physician and nursing care, drugs, medical supplies, therapeutic services, home health care, and nutrition counseling. It also will cover up to five days at a time of inpatient care as a respite for caregivers, although it will not pay for room and board in a hospital or nursing home. You can imagine what a relief such respite can be for you.

The patients must agree not to seek curative treatment for the terminal illness. They also waive their right to standard Medicare coverage for the terminal condition. (Unrelated health problems can still be attended to, though.) Medicare covers the cost of the services of the beneficiary's own physician, even if he/she is not on the hospice team. This applies to both traditional Medicare and to Medicare HMOs. Recipients may cancel the hospice benefit at any time and return to standard Medicare coverage. If they should need to sign up for hospice at a later time, that would also be possible.

Medicaid covers hospice in most states. Eligibility requirements and benefits are similar to Medicare's. Check with your state Medicaid office for further information. Private health plans also pay for some hospice care. Ask your provider for details.

If the patient is going to end his/her days in a facility rather than at home, you still have a right to hospice care, which is available regardless of where you are. If you're over sixty-five, you're entitled to a comprehensive hospice benefit. Your local hospice branch can give you further details. They're listed in the yellow pages of phone books.

There are different end-of-life concerns in a nursing home or a hospital: Will you be there at the last moment? Do you want to be there? Do you want to arrange for any last rites? Do you want to have anyone else at the bedside? If you want to be present, there are places that will allow you to sleep on a cot, next to the patient's bed, or in a nearby room. If you feel that being there at the moment of death is just too much for you to consider, that's OK, just act accordingly. After all, the person you knew and loved disappeared long ago in his/her dementia. You've been mourning that loss for what seems like forever. It's hard to even remember what the patient was like before the nightmare started. The memory will come back, though, little by little.

Inform the doctors and nurses in the facility what your wishes are about autopsy. There are those who are opposed to it on religious grounds, and there are those who fervently want an autopsy in order to have the diagnosis confirmed. Find an understanding professional within the facility, and sit down ahead of time to discuss the concerns you have and the directives you must share with them. The earlier you take care of things, the fewer burdensome details you will have to address at the time of death.

Try to decide ahead of time which funeral home you want. Avoid choosing the cemetery and gravesite at the last minute. It will surely cost you more, in money and stress. Speaking of cost, be prepared to spend thousands of dollars on funeral and burial arrangements. Have the money in your name only, since any joint assets may be temporarily frozen when the bank is notified by Social Security of the death. The funeral home is required to notify Social Security. Some of the expenses can be charged on a credit card, but some cannot. The cemetery I dealt with wanted no part of a charge card, and the funeral home needed some payment in the form of a check.

Although we have come a long way since the publication years ago of *The High Cost of Death and Dying*, different funeral homes charge different fees for the same services. You've been strong up until now, so do this one more thing to make yourself feel proud of yourself. Check out the different facilities. Don't hesitate to reject any wasteful or useless feature, no matter how strong the pressure. It might be possible to inquire on the phone. I did. Since Newton wanted a plain pine coffin with wooden pegs, there was no need to pick a casket, despite the pressure to do so coming from the first funeral home I was in touch with. If the deceased was a veteran, he/she can be buried in a military cemetery (a substantial savings) and is entitled to have an American flag draped over the coffin.

Even if you have prepaid arrangements, be sure to have some money set aside anyway since there can be uncovered charges you didn't know about. Newton's father had repeatedly told him that everything was taken care of. As it turned out, a limousine was paid for, but the fee for digging the grave was not. That can cost as much as the grave itself. There is the renting of the room for the ceremony if you don't want only a graveside service, and on and on.

Most people host a collation of some kind after the funeral. You need someone to set things out while you're still away, so that it can be waiting when you all come back to your house. That can be difficult, since most of the people you're close to and can trust with your keys will want to be at the funeral. Perhaps one funeral service attendee won't go to the cemetery, and he/she can help out. Or someone can host the collation in another home. You could also eat out.

Funeral homes are well equipped to deal with many of the details. They will send you as many death certificates as you want. Order more than you think you'll need, since official and financial transactions will require an original death certificate. Only a few places will accept a photocopy or send you back the original. Ordering the death certificate later on from the appropriate local government office is possible, but very slow.

Also through the funeral home you can arrange to have an obituary put into the newspaper of your choice. The advantages are obvious, but the disadvantages are not: obituaries tell the whole world that the person has died and that the family will be out of the house during the funeral. Unscrupulous con men read the obits to find potential victims for home repair or investment scams. They contact survivors and claim that the deceased put a deposit down on something, and then ask the survivor for the balance. The item in question was to be a surprise gift for you, and looks pretty good, especially through the veil of sentimentality. It's usually worthless, though.

Bank employees go through the obituaries to find out whether it is necessary to seal a safety deposit box. Boxes are sealed the minute a bank finds out one of the cosigners has died. It cannot be unsealed until the state tax department or some other authority issues permission. That sometimes requires a visit to the box by a tax representative. This can take many months. So, don't leave a will or any such vital document in the safety deposit box, or else be sure that you will absolutely be able to gain access to it before the person dies—hard to do on weekends or holidays.

Soon after the funeral, you will start to receive offers for gravestones. The monument people have been given your name by either the funeral home or the cemetery. Although you can contact them and shop around for prices, keep in mind that it's impossible to return a stone once it has been carved. So, be sure that the company you're dealing with is reputable. Ask for references, or better yet, ask people you know for referrals to places that gave them complete satisfaction. Insist on seeing a pattern of what the stone will look like before it is chiseled. Show it to your clergyman to make sure all is in order. Consider all the relationships of the deceased and list as many as you think are appropriate. The usual order is to put the spousal relationship first, followed by the parenting and grandparenting relationship, and then the roles of sibling, child, or friend your loved one held at the time of death.

It will be helpful to find out details about what Social Security can offer you. For example, you may be entitled to a $255 funeral benefit. It doesn't pay for the cost of the funeral, but it's a small help. If you are at least sixty years old, you might be entitled to widow/er's benefits. As for when Social Security reclaims its last payment, here's the explanation: A recipient is paid on the third of the month for having lived out the entire previous month. Therefore, if someone dies before the end of a month, the money that is given on the third of the following month is not rightfully the beneficiary's. It can come as a shock if the money is reclaimed, and that is all the more reason you must have some money set aside.

No matter what your religious convictions, there will be a lot of people surrounding you before, during, and after the funeral. People do care, they just don't always know how to show it or have the time to spare from their own busy schedules to give you extended periods of consolation. It is an especially good deed to call on someone recently bereaved after the crowds have left. That's when you feel your aloneness the most keenly. The silence echoes around you. The focus of your day-to-day activities is gone. There doesn't seem to be any real reason to get up in the morning. There's so much to attend to, it's bewildering. You just want to give up.

I believe a little self-pity is good. Allow yourself to wallow for a few days. Then you'll be better able to pick yourself up, dust yourself off, and start all over again.

CHECKLIST

- ❏ Should the patient end his/her days at home, in a nursing home or hospital, or in a hospice?
- ❏ If you want home hospice care, have a physician give you the referral ahead of time.
- ❏ Should there be an autopsy? What about organ donations?
- ❏ Which funeral home should you use? Which type of coffin will you choose? Will you ask for cremation? What are the religious requirements? Who should officiate? Do you want eulogies? If you do, select the speakers. Choose who will help you with food and other arrangements when the time comes. (You don't necessarily have to notify all these people, just have them set in your mind.)
- ❏ What signs and symptoms will you see before the death? Tell the medical professionals what you want in the way of information and support.

❑ Make sure you have a few thousand dollars readily available in your name alone, not in a joint account with the patient.

❑ Attend to any safe deposit boxes you have with the patient as cosigner: Empty the box, or leave in it only those things you can do without for a year.

❑ Know what to expect from Social Security. Call (800) 772-1213 for details.

❑ How many death certificates will you need? Have military discharge papers, if any, ready, along with a birth certificate, etc.

❑ Have a list of people to call, and decide who can take on some of the phone calling for you.

ADDITIONAL READING ABOUT DEATH AND DYING

Anderson, Patricia. *Affairs in Order.* New York: Collier/Macmillan, 1991.

Beresford, Larry. *The Hospice Handbook.* New York: Little, Brown and Co., 1993.

Hatch, Robert T. *How to Embalm Your Mother-in-Law.* Secaucus, N.J.: Citadel, 1993.

Knox, Jean McBee. *Death and Dying.* Broomall, Pa.: Chelsea House, 1989.

Young, Gregory W. *The High Cost of Dying.* Buffalo, N.Y.: Prometheus Books, 1994.

CHAPTER 8

A New Beginning

Now you are alone, with memories and doubts swirling around you. Little hopes and big fears occupy what free time you can squeeze in among all the paperwork and chores that can't be neglected any more. You're reluctant to look in the mirror; you barely recognize yourself. At least, when your loved one was still alive, you had a purpose to your day, if that was only to get through it.

This is the time to think about you. What would you really like to do (besides recapture the past, of course)? Are there any accomplishments you've fantasized about? Is there a skill you never had any time to develop? This is your chance. Sure, you have to attend to the legal, financial, and housekeeping demands. But those can't be allowed to occupy all your thoughts. No one will criticize you at this point. So take that trip, or do the unthinkable you've craved for so long.

Despite my encouraging you to do something special for yourself, I in no way want to give you the impression that there isn't a mourning period to go through. If you don't acknowledge a need to mourn and work through your sadness and anger, you will not heal. Yes, you can forget your grief temporarily, but years later, the underlying pain will linger and prevent you from being all you can be. There are many books on the mourning process, so there is no need to repeat the stages of mourning here. This is the place to talk about support groups, therapy, and healing. They will lead to a better tomorrow.

There is a wide choice of bereavement groups out there: hospitals, churches, senior centers, and mental health care centers might all have such a group. Most are funded through government or private donations, so you don't have to worry about another financial outlay. They meet during the day or in the evening. They accept the recently bereaved or insist on a wait of a few months. It's up to you to track down what will meet your needs. It won't be a hard search, since all the leaders of such groups really want to be helpful and want a variety of members to join. There is one requirement, though: you must commit to coming for a set number of weeks. Most groups meet once a week, and missing a session makes your growth and the group's cohesion more difficult. So, if you've already booked that passage on a tour around the world, don't sign up just yet for a bereavement support group.

Why even join such a group to begin with? Isn't time the best healer? Besides, you don't want to hear other people's problems: you have enough of your own sadness, and all that won't bring back your loved one. But until you try it and visit a bereavement group, you won't know how truly beneficial it can be to share grief, and believe it or not, share a few good laughs with others who are in a similar situation. Seeing that others feel as you do, fear many of the same fears, and desire some of the same apparently unattainable goals is a tremendous consolation. I have known a great many survivors of mourning. Those who seem to be most able to live a serene life are those who have had some kind of bereavement counseling. As a matter of fact, I was surprised to learn of how many participated in more than one support group. They signed up with a new support group after their first series was over. They felt they needed more time to process their grief, and they were wise enough to make the opportunity to do so.

Consider private, individual counseling as well. A loss of someone close to you, especially after a long illness during which you helplessly watch him/her degenerate, brings all sorts of buried issues close to the surface. You may be terrified that you will end up like the one you've lost, a burden, a helpless shadow of yourself. Now is your chance to work on those fears and on the many other issues that have been neglected over the years. That, too, will help you heal. Ask your doctor for a referral to a competent therapist. If you know someone who has made strides thanks to counseling, ask for the name of the therapist. If you think you can't afford to pay, seek out mental health clinics. They usually have a sliding pay scale. Look in your phone book. Although the competence of the therapist is important, you are the one who must do the hard work, so even a beginner counselor under adequate supervision can offer you cleansing and progress.

Seeing a private therapist doesn't interfere with the discussions in a bereavement group. As a matter of fact, one can complement the other. You can even use some of your reactions in the group as a jumping-off point for a private session. I would urge you not to give up the group, where you will meet others and take those first steps in human relationships as a solo in a safe and supportive environment.

One of the benefits of participating in a bereavement support group is the development of friendships with other group members. You can hit it off with someone and share outside activities and conversations. Friendship is always important, but it is crucial at a time of loss and loneliness. These new friends cannot supplant your old ones, but they can add an enriching dimension to your interests and activities. Your old friends will be somewhat relieved, as a matter of fact, to hear that you are moving on with your life. Your company will be more desirable, since they won't fear that they will be called upon to console you endlessly. While you're at it, weed out the friends who have made you feel uncomfortable for quite a while. If you're angry at them for not being there when you most needed them, tell them so. Let them present their side. Don't make hasty judgments, but don't hesitate to satisfy your needs, either.

Friendships are one thing, but what about romance? Are you available? If so, maybe one of the group members is just your type. If you have lost your sweetheart, you miss that closeness and intimacy you had with the deceased. There are times you think you would do anything to recapture some moments, some special feelings. The problem is, you are exceedingly needy. If your potential partner was recently widowed, he/she may also be exceptionally needy, whether he/she is in a support group or not. You don't really want to be used as a bandage to cover a wound, do you? When that wound heals, the bandage is discarded. Nor would you want to be in the position of discarding someone you would feel you had outgrown. There will be joys and disappointments in new romance. Why put yourself under unnecessary pressure while you're still dealing with active mourning? You know that a song, a smell, the turn of someone's head, will make you cry for your lost beloved.

So, if you are widowed, try to develop friendships. You can grow and heal with their companionship. However, I would advise you to avoid becoming romantically involved for many months. A year is a nice round number to set as your goal for being ready to "get out there." Give yourself permission to grieve. You will be a more complete person for doing so. After a year, all the holidays and anniversaries will have passed one time, and you will know in the depth of your being that you can survive. There's nothing like feeling worthy to make you a desirable love partner.

What kind of activities can you participate in? There are some, like dancing, that are difficult to engage in without a partner (although you could take a line dance class, or go to a ballroom setting in which people just dance, for the fun of it). But a great variety of activities can be done alone, even ones you would never have considered doing on your own in the past. Have you attended a show, seen a movie, gone to a concert by yourself? If not, give it a try. You may be pleasantly surprised. Look into adult education courses. They offer subjects ranging from business classes to painting and physical fitness. Physical exercise provides a wonderful release from tension. If one center doesn't have what you want or the classes don't meet at a convenient time, try another. Community colleges are another source for a large variety of courses.

Decisions, decisions . . . Will you need to go to work? Do you want to, even just to be part of a structured environment that pays on a regular basis? You might still be working, as you were during your entire ordeal. Do you now want to explore other career opportunities? If you hesitate because of your age, remember that there have been people who got their first college degree in their late eighties. In five years, you'll be five years older whether or not you've done what you really wanted to do. Why not make the birthday celebration more complete?

If you don't want a job but would like to have some commitments that will give you flexibility with your time, consider volunteering with an organization of your choice. We tend to think of hospitals when we think of being a volunteer. While those are great sources for a variety of volunteer positions, there are many other opportunities. You can work in an airport as a Travelers Aid volunteer, or teach reading in a youth home. Look in the newspaper, where there are sometimes ads from organizations that specialize in placing volunteers. Even if you don't know exactly what you would like to do, they can interview you and make suggestions. Senior centers may also have leads.

If your family now sees you as a great source for free babysitting, repairs, cooking, or whatever, it's up to you to set limits on how much you want to do. If spending time with your grandchildren is the greatest boost to your morale, go for it. But if you want a breather or a change of pace, you will feel trapped unless you've entered into previous agreements outlining details of your commitment and your availability. I'm a great believer in written agreements between friends and family as well as with contractors. Such an agreement forces both parties to clarify their understanding of the relationship. It becomes a neutral source of reference should any questions arise. Most of all, it makes sure each participant knows what's expected of him/her.

Family can now be your greatest support, or your greatest frustration, much as they were during your loved one's illness. Little by little, everyone goes back to familiar roles and activities. If there are grudges, clear them up. You will be listened to more now than at any other time. You have more perspective, as well as greater needs. Think of how you would like to be remembered when your time comes. Clearing out old emotional cobwebs is good for the soul and helps the healing process. Decide how important a slight really is, and act accordingly. Tell loved ones around you that you love them. See what happens.

What if you have no family? What if your family is distant, physically and otherwise? Here is your chance to create a family. Friends cannot take the place of relatives, but they are chosen. Adopt a sibling, if only in your mind. When you give of yourself, the gesture comes back to warm you sooner or later. Look into your religious affiliation. Houses of worship offer a family-like structure that can be most supportive, if only because of their traditions. They also present you with an opportunity to participate in a choice of activities, be they social or charitable. Both will contribute to your feelings of accomplishment and well-being (or should I say "better-being"?).

If your family is far away, and you'd like to be closer, you might be tempted to move. You might also want to get out of a home where there are so many sad memories. Hold off. You don't want to act on something as drastic as leaving your home when you're in a vulnerable position. Again, wait a year. You will see things much more clearly by then. After a year, it may still be time to make the move. But now you will be uprooting yourself after careful thinking and planning rather than out of desperation. Part of the mourning process is finding out what works for you, from eating breakfast out to moving across the continent.

Being newly bereaved is truly a case of half empty: You are now half of what you were, the survivor of a partnership, whether it be with a spouse or other loved one. But it is also a case of seeing the glass half full. This terribly sad time is an opportunity for growth, exploration, and inner enrichment. It's all in how you look at it. Choose to see how you can develop, and your future will gradually shape up as a bright one.

CHECKLIST

- ❑ Make a list of things you would really like to do. Pick one of those things and do it.

- ❑ Locate a bereavement support group appropriate for your needs. Sign up for it, even if it isn't scheduled to start for quite a while.

- ❑ Line up the name of a competent therapist, if you should need one.

- ❑ Clear up old grudges. Apologize even if you don't remember for sure it was your fault.

- ❑ Decide what kind of relationship you would like to have with different family members. Meet with them and share your thoughts where appropriate.

- ❑ Make an effort to befriend someone. Keep in contact with your old friends, especially to tell them something positive.

- ❑ Do one thing alone that you have never done alone.

- ❑ Find out about jobs or job training or volunteer work that is to your liking.

- ❑ Ask friends or family what, if anything, they would like you to do for them. Then write out the terms of your arrangement.

- ❑ Explore the advantages of your religion's institutions. Allow yourself to become part of that community.

SUGGESTED ADDITIONAL READING
ABOUT LIVING ON YOUR OWN

Finley, Mitch. *101 Ways to Nourish Your Soul.* New York: Crossroad Publishing Co., 1996.

Grant, Wendy. *Are You in Control?* Rockport, Mass.: Element Books, 1996.

Hall, Doug. *Making the Courage Connection.* New York: Fireside Books, 1997.

Helmstetter, Shad. *Choices.* New York: Pocket Books, 1989.

CHAPTER 9

The Child Speaks

The child of a person with Alzheimer's or other forms of dementia has special issues to deal with. They are varied and complex. Here is a sampling of interviews with sons and daughters of these parents who have disappeared into a world of their own. It is hoped that these children's words will both console and advise. The names used are pseudonyms.

▷ Carl is a man over forty whose mother had died three months before the interview, three years after she was diagnosed with Alzheimer's.

QUESTION: What was the hardest part of seeing your mother go through the changes involved in Alzheimer's?
ANSWER: The fact that she was aware that she was losing her mind, and in her lucid moments would cry about it. She knew she was going into a darkness from which there was no return. She suffered even more because of the humiliation: there was some awareness; there had to be. Why else did she constantly rip off the diapers? The physical stuff was also hard, her incontinence and seeing her play with her feces on the wall. She had always been so fastidious! I would go and have to clean her up. My stepfather would call me to do it. Then I got him a helper. I just brought her to the door, and he hired her. In my mother's mind, she herself was still doing the things she always did, like cleaning the house, which was really filthy and smelly.

I couldn't help her. I could just play the piano and sing songs. We sang to the end. She would remember lyrics from the forties. She would get into it and act and be coquettish. She had been a beautiful woman. I'll tell you a strange thing: I taught her a new song a year and a half into her illness, and she remembered it until the end, when she couldn't sing or talk, except to say "Ow" if something hurt her. It's incredible. That's why music is so far-reaching, it just gets into your soul.

Another difficult part is when she turned on me and said nasty things. They were filthy and hurtful things. It stabbed me like a knife when she told me she was sorry that she ever had me. She had been a manic-depressive person with delusional and paranoid moments, a victim of the cruelty that her stepmother inflicted on her. (But she was a loving woman.) So I expected her to have a tough old age, but I wasn't ready for Alzheimer's. It was horrific to see the strongest one in the family fall apart.

QUESTION: Was there a role reversal? How did you feel about it?
ANSWER: Yes, absolutely, but we had a role reversal my whole life because she never knew what to do. I was prepared and therefore not so upset by it. I was used to it and felt that this was my calling. And I felt confident making decisions for her because I knew her best. My father just wanted to be left alone while I was growing up. Her loss of physical control made her a child. She was childlike mentally, too: she would ask a question ten times. The only way to deal with it was to assume that this was my child. That happened because I loved this person.

QUESTION: Was there any positive outcome from this experience?
ANSWER: No. I loved her before, and I may have told her I loved her more when she was sick, but she didn't remember. Actually, I'm a lot like my mother, and it's scary. If it's true that Alzheimer's is hereditary, I'm scared.

QUESTION: Were you often angry? At what? How did you handle your anger or sadness?

ANSWER: I wasn't often angry, because my anger toward Mom was worked out before, when I became an adult. And I wasn't angry at the powers that be. I knew that my mother was going to be sick some day. That's why I know (and knew it before the disease) that I want to work out all emotional problems before old age.

I'm angry at my stepfather because he is a non-active person. He could have done more. But he dealt with her and paid for the basics, even though he wouldn't pay for the air conditioning.

As for sadness, I handled it by crying. I cry easily; I'm not against men crying.

QUESTION: How did others around you relate to the patient and to you?

ANSWER: I had battles with my brother because he wanted to put her in a home right away, disgusted by my stepfather's inactions. But I kept her at home because I knew how afraid my mother was. And I myself want to die at home. My brother and stepfather just wanted to be done with it "so we don't have to suffer with it so much." So I ruled, with my stepfather's approval. But they wanted expediency rather than what was best for Mother. They annoyed me and second-guessed me many times. It bothered me because I like to get along with my family.

QUESTION: Were you given adequate information about the progression of the disease at the outset? If not, would it have helped if you had? How were the health care professionals you dealt with?

ANSWER: No, I was not given adequate information. Yes, it would have helped if I had, because more information always helps, but I don't know that I would have done things differently. We dealt with the progression of the disease as we went along. And I knew some details from the psychiatrist when my mother was committed to the psychiatric ward of a hospital. But he didn't call to ask how she was doing, and the other doctors were cold. The caregivers need tenderness and caring, and the medical people don't give it to them. The health care professionals only did the minimum, what they had to do.

They didn't tell us the full story about my mother's situation after she fell and broke her hip, either. In the hospital, my brother and I were told that she had to have a hip replacement operation, or else she would be bedridden for the rest of her life. She would also suffer pain while the bones were setting incorrectly. We didn't think to ask questions, didn't know what questions to ask. We gave permission for the operation. What no one mentioned was the fact that you have to go to rehab and learn to walk again after this operation. You can't learn to walk, or anything else for that matter, when your mind is ravaged by Alzheimer's disease. So my mother was bedridden anyway. And do you think the surgery and healing were painless? To make matters worse, after the hip replacement, it became infected and twisted. They removed the artificial hip and left her a pretzel. After that second operation, she had a feeding tube and a catheter and deep bed sores.

I wanted her not to be put on a respirator when she got pneumonia, but her husband overruled me. She did smile once or twice, but I don't know whether it was worth it to her.

QUESTION: What mistakes did you make?
ANSWER: I blame myself for her getting the hip replacement and for not having asked more questions and raised more objections. The woman taking care of her called me to ask for shorter blankets because my mother would get tangled up in hers, but I didn't get the blanket fast enough, and my mother tripped because she was entangled in the blanket. That's when she broke her hip.

She just got worse even faster after breaking the hip. But is that a bad thing? I sometimes fantasized about ending her life. . . . And I wonder whether I should have taken her in when my father died, because I was the closest to her.

QUESTION: What are you most proud of?
ANSWER: I was most proud of telling her that I loved her as much

as I did; it felt as good for me as for her. We fought a lot, and I over-came my anger toward her to tell her I loved her. Also, I gave her such joy through music.

QUESTION: What advice would you give the child of an Alzheimer's parent at the outset of the disease? Near the end?

ANSWER: I wouldn't give any advice, except to read as much as possible and contact the Alzheimer's Association. It is such a personal thing. Just be prepared for anything and get as much help as you can. And try to get the family to be open with one another and pull together to attack the situation. It is much easier for the caregivers if they are together in solidarity. And it would help the patient, too: they hear you more than you think. They're there, they just can't remember. But they are there, and should be treated as such. They know when you are arguing about whether to put them in a home or not.

QUESTION: What financial advice would you give?

ANSWER: Financially, I would say you have to use common sense, get the most help for the most amount of money you can afford.

QUESTION: Is there anything you would like to add?

ANSWER: There was relief when she passed, but you miss even the aggravation. Now I remember her as she was and that is how I miss her.

▷   Jane is a woman past thirty-five. She works full time. Her job keeps her in contact with many people, usually on a one-to-one basis. Her mother, who was diagnosed with Alzheimer's six years ago, still lives in her own home. Jane moved back in with her mother at first, but found that the pressure of caregiving and working was too much for her. A year ago, her mother's care became the responsibility of one of Jane's sisters.

Before the diagnosis, the family began to notice suspicious symptoms. The first change was the mother's reaction to her retirement: she seemed to lose track of time and be forgetful. Since she had worked nights for years, her children thought the shift to daytime activity and the normal aging process were responsible for their mother's change in behavior. Then she seemed to be a bit more confused when her close friend moved away. When uncharacteristic behavior developed, especially having to do with money, the children could no longer ignore the symptoms. They had their mother tested.

QUESTION: What is the hardest part of seeing your mother go through the changes involved in Alzheimer's?

ANSWER: Seeing her be in and out of it and try to hide it and be very weepy. If only she could "go over" and not know, it would be better. She thought she was losing her mind and was trying to describe it. She was obsessed with calendars. She had fifteen around her, but it didn't help. Also, she would just come in in the middle of the night and start asking me questions. I had no privacy.

No more now that she has "gone over." She goes to a group she loves, and she is better than the others, but it's sad to see her in that situation. They're like little children, throwing balls.

I was living with her when she was diagnosed, and now I live forty minutes away, and that's better. My other family members took over, and I don't see her that often. She's at home.

Why don't I go more often? Because I started to have anxiety attacks. It took a bigger toll on me than I realized.

QUESTION: Is there a role reversal? How do you feel about it?

ANSWER: Yes. It was weird. She resented it, too, even though it had to be that way. It was about my being a parent to a rebellious teenager. She put together some strange outfits to wear, and then she started to ask me for help picking clothes to go together when she would go to the group. My sister bought her new outfits and that worked. Since I don't live with her any more, my contact with her is kept very light and social, and there isn't that tension. My siblings feel that tension now. But they don't resent my having moved away, since they knew I needed to move after five years. At first I resisted having them take over.

The sister who is now the caregiver and I had probably the worst relationship with my mother. So my sister should be prepared for attacks. She thought she could do it for a year. It was better than it was for me, but it is very draining for my sister. But she kept her own apartment, and so she has a place of retreat to go to. Since I have six sisters and one brother, someone would take my mother for the weekend. When I was living with her, my mother didn't want to leave home, because it was disorienting to go elsewhere. Now, because her disease has progressed, she is more willing to go and is more cooperative. We also make sure that she always has ID on her and that she carries a key.

QUESTION: Are you often angry? At what? How do you handle it? What about sadness?

ANSWER: Yes, I have been angry because my mother resented what I was doing instead of appreciating it. After a year away, I've worked it out. I was in counseling and I still am.

As for sadness: I used to get really upset about her confused state, when she was trying to figure things out. She always was a difficult, controlling person, but once she started to accept it a little more, we could talk about it and cry together about her losing control over her life.

Before that, instead of blaming the illness when her driver's license was taken away, she blamed me. It was my fault. She used to forget when I used to tell her where I was going, and then she would call someone to say I had simply left, with no explanation. She would dramatize things, saying I had run out of the house, and that simply was not true. Then I learned to write notes, and that helped. One of my sisters my mother used to call at such times now realizes what the real situation was, that it wasn't me.

Slowly, people caught on. When she was staying with my sister for the weekend, she would call me to complain! She would concoct a story rather than just ask to go home. My sister Karen saw that when she went walking with a friend for just an hour, that was what my mother would focus on and ignore all the other attention. Then my sister saw my situation more clearly.

QUESTION: How do others relate to the patient? To you?

ANSWER: At the beginning, a lot of people wouldn't believe she had Alzheimer's. She would be very personable and she could follow a conversation. People thought she should be totally gone. But if they were around for an extended period of time, they would see the repetitive nature of her behavior. Then they started to worry about their own parents. But they were very sympathetic. It touches on everybody's fear that it can happen to them or to a loved one. One of my sisters was thinking that she had Alzheimer's, and that was triggering things, too. I told her that her forgetfulness was just stress.

We started to clean out the garage in case we would have to sell the house. Phase one could last from one to seven years. But my mother collected bags of things and piled them up in the garage all over again. This is what she does all day long, packing stuff. She was putting away the weirdest things, like a vacuum cleaner attachment.

QUESTION: Were you given adequate information about the progression of the disease at the outset?

ANSWER: Not really. I find that her doctors didn't know that much about it. But the group that she was in through the Alzheimer's foundation told my sister a lot. And I read books about it.

It would have been a help if I had been told more. They would diagnose by process of elimination, so they tried a medication and said to wait for four months for the results. I wanted to try a holistic route, but the rest of the family didn't.

A neurologist was the best person in her HMO. Her general doctor said, when her driver's license was taken away, "Just let her drive until she runs out of gas." Imagine! The medication she was on was making her lose her appetite, and she was withering away and nauseous all the time. So he said to take her off for a week, load her with junk food to fatten her up, and then put her back on! So I kept her on the medication until this new stuff came out. Just the pill taking alone could drive you crazy! It had to be taken at just the right time, and she wouldn't know if she had taken it. The second medication didn't affect her appetite, but it did no good. She may still be taking it, I don't know.

Then the general doctor put her on an antidepressant and that became another pill that she had to take and it didn't help her, so she came off of it. My mother liked this guy. My sister took her to the doctor because of my work schedule, and she liked him, too.

Anything my mother heard on TV she wanted to do, like estrogen therapy, or taking ibuprofen or vitamin E. Nothing seemed to help anyway.

QUESTION: What are you most proud of?
ANSWER: That I didn't lose my mind [laugh]. Someone I know, who was on Prozac, said anyone taking care of an Alzheimer's patient has to have a nervous breakdown. I never lost my temper with my mother. I think my meditation helped me to try to stay focused. She would ask me a hundred times what day it was, and I would just tell her. My sister Karen wouldn't put up with that. My mother took advantage of my nature.

I had a lot of support from friends. I maintained my own life, and that's the thing that allowed me not to have that kind of resentment. My mother would try to help me cook, and she would put things away when I needed them, and so on. She tried cooking and it tasted awful. She burned out the microwave because she would put things in and forget about them. That scared her and then she would just make tea. I learned to cook large portions and freeze the food, so I didn't have to cook every night.

The interactions with my different sisters have brought most of us closer, except for my oldest sister. She would disagree with everything because she wanted the control of the money, but she didn't want to take care of my mother. She is the oldest and I am the youngest. She finally stopped because it made life too difficult for me and I told her. She wanted the control of making Mother's medical appointments. She expected her siblings to take Mother without consulting them about the time. We used to have family meetings and it would flare up. Then she refused to come to any more meetings, so she is not in contact with any of us. It was when she found out that she, the oldest, was not the executrix that she became like that. It was all about the money.

QUESTION: What mistakes have you made?
ANSWER: The doctor thing: I should have been more adamant about finding a doctor who knew more about Alzheimer's. That medication drove me crazy. The neurologist told us to take her off the medication in four months, but it didn't help any and they kept her on it so long.

I can't decide if it was a mistake to go back and move in with my mother. I had to move out of where I lived, my mother wanted to sell her house, and my sister from California wanted to buy it a year later. I thought maybe we could patch up our relationship and bond in one year. It was a fantasy. My sister in California didn't come and my mother was diagnosed with Alzheimer's.

We had to switch everything over because of Medicaid. Then there was a three-year wait on that, and that is now over. So now we should put her in a place that deals with Alzheimer's patients. My mother didn't want to go into a home, but we are considering it now. I brought in a cat, and my mother became attached to him, he became her buddy. She would say, "What will I do with Buddy?" Today I can't have a conversation with her about such decisions. Family meetings with all of us, including Mother, to discuss the will, the proxies, etc., became very awkward. But we went through it, and it was a relief when it was done because we know how she felt about things.

QUESTION: Does going to work help?
ANSWER: Yes, it takes me out of that whole environment and gives me other things to do. And I have met others who had people with Alzheimer's, and they have been helpful.

QUESTION: What advice would you give the child of a parent who was recently diagnosed with Alzheimer's?

ANSWER: Don't live with the person if at all possible. Get in touch with Alzheimer organizations right away and get as much information as possible. A support group is great, if you can go to one.

QUESTION: What financial advice would you like to give?

ANSWER: I wish we had done that switchover stuff ahead of time.

▷ Jeff's father was diagnosed with dementia, and died of congestive heart failure suffered after a broken neck three years after the diagnosis. He had been a diabetic and had had a series of minor strokes that no one had been aware of until the damage was done.

QUESTION: What was the hardest part of seeing your father go through the changes involved in dementia?

ANSWER: Just seeing him weakened to the point where he became someone different from the father I remembered.

QUESTION: Was there a role reversal?

ANSWER: Yes, but my parents lived far from me, so I would go down and spend a weekend to relieve my mother. He was incontinent at the end, and I took care of that, so that was definitely a role reversal. I felt sad, frustrated, angry, and scared of being unable to handle the situation physically and emotionally. The only thing that was an issue at the end was how I felt. It was sad, just because he was my father. We were always buddies. That's the good part: it was a complete relationship, and there isn't anything I think I should have said but didn't. There is nothing I regret, up to the end.

QUESTION: Was there any positive outcome from this experience?

ANSWER: For my mother there was because his death freed her to fulfill herself for the rest of her life, which she is in the process of doing. He just wouldn't allow himself to enjoy life, even when he was able to financially. He felt he didn't deserve anything. The dementia brought about a chance for the two of them to feel a closeness that they never had. They were married fifty years minus two months.

QUESTION: Were you often angry? At what? How did you handle your anger or sadness?
ANSWER: I wasn't often angry, but it was part of what I was dealing with emotionally. I was angry at him because he didn't take care of himself when he was healthy and so he put himself in that situation. I tried to ignore the anger, look at it unemotionally. Then I realized that the anger isn't going to help and then I let it go. I meditate. But the sadness is here to stay.

QUESTION: How did others around you relate to the patient and to you?
ANSWER: Some of the relatives paid a little more attention to him than they had before. There was no change in the way they dealt with me.

QUESTION: Were you given adequate information about the progression of the disease at the outset? How were the health care professionals you dealt with?
ANSWER: No, we were not given adequate information. He was misdiagnosed a lot. The bad part is that by the time they found a doctor who could treat him, it was too late. My experience seeing my parents get older is that geriatric patients don't get good care. The doctors do what they want to, don't give them credence, and are insensitive to them.

It would have helped me a little bit if I had been informed. Maybe things would have made a little more sense.

The health care professionals I met were good. Two or three women came a few times a week and they were very good. They relieved my mother and gave her a break to get out.

It was difficult because my father wouldn't stay down, and he was so unsteady that he would fall all the time. He was bruised and bloody frequently. That part was very difficult. He understood, but he just wasn't going to sit around waiting until he was dead. He wanted to do things, even if he had to suffer the consequences.

QUESTION: What mistakes did you make?
ANSWER: At the beginning, when I was angry with him, that was a mistake. But I didn't show it to him. We were always friends. I step back rather than releasing my anger. But this is a normal reaction to a horrible situation. So it wasn't really a mistake.

QUESTION: What are you most proud of?
ANSWER: My mother: she just did a good job taking care of him. It was hard, but she gave him love.

QUESTION: What advice would you give the child of a dementia patient at the outset of the disease, and at the end?
ANSWER: At the outset, try to remember the fact that you were an infant once and that this person took good care of you then. I'd give the same advice at the end of the illness, too.

QUESTION: What financial advice would you give?
ANSWER: Be a good bookkeeper when you're dealing with all the agencies. Consider how to handle what money there is, or you could lose it all.

▷ Fred lives with his mother who was diagnosed with Alzheimer's four or five years ago. He has two brothers, but he is her primary caregiver. He has had the help of an aide for the past nine months. She stays with his mother while he goes to his demanding job. Unfortunately, his mother won't let anyone but him bathe her, and she still doesn't recognize the aide's name. He says, embarrassed, "How can I be giving my mother a bath?" His mother has unpredictable ups and downs but consistently cannot write her own name.

Fred takes his mother to various functions associated with work, and few people realize that behind her still-pretty smile lies emptiness. His entire schedule centers around his mother's needs. His deep religious beliefs give him strength.

QUESTION: What is the hardest part of seeing your mother go through the changes involved in Alzheimer's?

ANSWER: It's letting go because she isn't anything like what I remember her to be. I let go piece by piece as she doesn't remember more and more. Now she doesn't remember family.

She's suffering from depression. That's very hard to deal with because she cries so much. When we changed the medication it was better, but now it's worse again. It's better if we go out in public, but she will not go out with the aide. There are nights that she doesn't sleep through completely, and now she doesn't always want to go to bed.

As it was happening, over the years, she didn't acknowledge her fears. Actually, she did, just once. She said, "This is about a bad dream." She might have been protecting me, not wanting to be a burden. Now, any time I ask her how she is, she always says that she has a cold. So she somehow knows something is wrong.

The really hard part is that you know that the only thing that is going to happen is that she will get worse. The question is what gets shut down next. I know I might inherit this. I just hope I die in my sleep.

Only as a last resort do I want to put her in a nursing home, if she needed it, or I just couldn't function.

QUESTION: Was there a role reversal? How did you feel about it?

ANSWER: Absolutely, there was a role reversal. She is like a child less than two years old. There is no adult left now. She can't make a logical sentence. If she were left alone for five minutes, she would get herself into trouble. When she understands anything, you have to be surprised and pleased.

In the beginning, I felt uncomfortable with it and resented it, but now I'm adjusted to it. I have two brothers. I think they are more uncomfortable because they still expect to see what she was. One brother lives out of state. But I don't ask my brother who is not so far away to watch her, I ask neighbors.

I am not myself. I have two lives, hers and work.

QUESTION: Are you often angry? At what? How do you handle it? What about sadness?

ANSWER: No, I'm not often angry. I'm not an angry person. Occasionally, though, on a bad day, I say, "I hate my life and I hate my job."

As for sadness, the things that got me sad at the beginning no longer affect me. Sometimes she says something that is enough of the mother I knew that it does affect me. She sometimes says, "You don't love me." If I'm OK, I soothe her, but if not, I say, "Do you think I would be doing this if I didn't love you?!" If I raise my voice it alarms her and is counterproductive.

QUESTION: How do others around you relate to your mother? To you?

ANSWER: People either think they can say "Do you remember me?" to her, and she has recall, or they have nothing to do with her because they have no understanding.

Toward me, people are generally understanding and compassionate. One of my brothers has been coming twice a year. We speak every week, and he and his wife are supportive, but his help is nonexistent. The brother who lives in my city cares, but is no help at all. He visited for twenty minutes last night after a three-week absence. He can't deal with it. Usually I don't resent it, but some days I do. I have accepted my brothers for who they are.

QUESTION: Were you given adequate information about the progression of the disease at the outset?

ANSWER: The neurologist who tested her didn't even have the decency to tell me the outcome. The internist never told me because he thought the neurologist told me. A year later, the doctor referred to Alzheimer's and that was the first I heard the word used in reference to my mother. The doctors I have dealt with never told me anything. I read everything that I know. I am informed, but not because it was given to me. I found other ways.

QUESTION: How were the health care professionals you dealt with?

ANSWER: The people I deal with now are kind and understanding. But they weren't particularly helpful at the beginning, not giving me suggestions. I found out everything on my own by accident.

QUESTION: What are you most proud of?
ANSWER: That we can make it through the day. Or now, it's more getting through an hour or a minute.

QUESTION: What mistakes have you made?
ANSWER: I don't know. I don't have any guilt. I haven't done anything terrible in choosing her health care. I forgive others, and I forgive myself, too.

QUESTION: Does going to work help?
ANSWER: Yes. Being with her requires a hundred percent of my attention and commitment. You are always on, even when you are sleeping. But work is an escape.

QUESTION: What advice would you give the child of a parent who was recently diagnosed with Alzheimer's?
ANSWER: Find out as much as you can, and enjoy as much as you can, while you still can. Have rough plans in your mind about what you will do next. For example, think about help at home versus nursing home care.

QUESTION: What financial advice would you like to give?
ANSWER: My mother kept everything in her name and I allowed her to let things stay that way to maintain her independence. But now I see that was a mistake. It didn't protect her or help her. If I had it to do over again, I would see a lawyer at the beginning.

Because I have lived with my mother for more than two years and I take care of her, Medicaid rules allow her house to be transferred to my name and they can't touch her assets. But the estate gift tax still applies.

▷ Yolanda and her husband, Harvey, are both over fifty-five. Her mother died five years before the interview. She was at first diagnosed with what the doctor called "dementia," and then with Alzheimer's. She lived six years after the diagnosis, the last three of which were spent in a nursing home. Both Yolanda and Harvey suspected it was Alzheimer's long before it was diagnosed because the mother reversed her right and left shoes and wore other people's glasses. The full-blown symptoms showed themselves at the time of a physical illness.

QUESTION: What was the hardest part of seeing your mother (and mother-in-law) go through the changes involved in her disease? **ANSWER:** It didn't bother me when she couldn't recognize me, but when she stopped talking even if it didn't make sense, that bothered me. Before that, when she would repeat the same questions time after time, my five-year-old grandson summed it up when he said, "That is the forgettingest lady."

The meanness she showed in the earlier stage was hard to deal with: she would explode suddenly and get mean with one of her great grandchildren, with no provocation. And she loved them!

QUESTION: Was there a role reversal? How did you feel about it? **ANSWER:** I guess there was a role reversal, but I never physically had to take care of her. She moved to an adult facility from her old apartment, and we hired a private person to help her, starting when she needed help taking her medication. She would either not take it, or she would take it too often.

HARVEY: I was expecting the deterioration. It happened very naturally. She would only stay here for a few days, for a weekend, and she would be like a tail and follow us all over the place. If Yolanda said that she was going downstairs to the basement, her mother would be looking for her hysterically.

She felt unfamiliar wherever she was. She would be so edgy when she came to visit, she wanted to go home after five minutes. So eventually we just switched to going to see her, bringing the grandchildren along.

It was a challenge to figure out how to deal with the various situations that came up, like the times she would misplace the TV remote or not even remember what the remote was for.

It was also hard to figure out how to handle the fact that her skin had become so sensitive.

QUESTION: Was there any positive outcome from this experience?
ANSWER: There isn't any. Just don't live too long; it's more hurtful. I often think of the *Star Trek* episode in which you are put to sleep after your sixty-fifth birthday party.

QUESTION: Were you often angry?
ANSWER: No, because we weren't living with her all the time. That was the saving grace for us. There was always a lot of sadness, especially when she couldn't communicate. When she died, she had been dead to me long before. There had been no interaction at the end. I no longer had a mother. Her death was a release. The end had finally come.

QUESTION: How did others around you relate to the patient and to you?
ANSWER: Verbally they were understanding and expressed sympathy, but privately they were tickled pink it wasn't them. No one knows really how it is unless you go through it.

It affects the whole family. I remember what happened with my oldest daughter: she didn't live far from the nursing home, and I would meet her there. She would start to cry, so I told her not to go any more, but just to remember her grandmother the way she used to be. And she stopped going. We didn't want the great-grand-children to remember her like that, either.

QUESTION: Were you given adequate information about the progression of the disease at the outset?
ANSWER: I don't think so. They asked questions before taking her into different facilities, but nobody told us what to expect. They tried to be supportive, though. My brother is a doctor and he

knew some of the nurses on the floor of the nursing home, so I think they were nicer because of that.

QUESTION: What mistakes did you make?
ANSWER: Not making the moves we had to make soon enough. You start thinking about these things while there is some understanding, and the person says they don't want to go there, so you back off. But you need hard love.

QUESTION: What are you most proud of?
ANSWER: Probably that everything that had to be done was done. There were no conflicts whatsoever within the family. My brother and I each paid half the expenses. We would try to go visit her together so we could talk to each other, not just stare at her.

QUESTION: What advice would you give the child of an Alzheimer's patient at the outset of the disease, and near the end?
ANSWER: At the outset, find out all that you can so you can be prepared. But sometimes you are better off not knowing, if you are going to become depressed and dysfunctional. Near the end, be sure there is a living will.

QUESTION: What financial advice would you give?
ANSWER: It is going to eat up everything you have. We didn't have a way to protect ourselves. We never used Medicaid, we paid for her and she thought that she still had enough money left to pay.

QUESTION: Is there anything you would like to add?
ANSWER: Yes. Somebody should find a cure. Hopefully this disease will disappear, the way polio disappeared years ago. I'm scared that I will develop Alzheimer's.

▷ Belle is over forty-five. Her father died nine months before the interview, after a ten-year illness. The diagnosis that he had "some sort of dementia" was changed to Alzheimer's disease after he had open-heart surgery.

QUESTION: What was the hardest part of seeing your father go through the changes involved in his disease?

ANSWER: Mentally he wasn't there any more. He didn't talk much. The last time I really spoke to him in a normal conversation was the eve of his open-heart surgery. He recuperated from the surgery, but he never came back to himself. He had been a strong, dynamic man who helped other people a lot. We used to laugh off the bizarre things he did, and then cry. I went into therapy at that point because he had been my best friend and my support. The therapist taught me that every day is another death.

QUESTION: Was there a role reversal? How did you feel about it?

ANSWER: Yes, there was. I felt that payback wasn't going to be that intense and extreme. But he was always there for me, so I became a sandwich generation. I knew it was my place to help my mother in life, so I didn't mind. It turned life around and I became very independent.

QUESTION: Was there any positive outcome from this experience?

ANSWER: The only positive outcome was that I became a stronger person.

QUESTION: Were you often angry?

ANSWER: Not really. I was too sad to be angry, I missed him too much while I was with him. He was in the nursing home two and a half years before he died. My sister and I put him in because we didn't want to lose our mother, too. He never wandered, but one day he hit her hard, and we decided to put him into a hospital and then into a nursing home.

QUESTION: How did others around you relate to your father and to you?

ANSWER: People close to us totally accepted the situation and visited a lot, but his colleagues stopped calling. His brothers and sisters would come to take him out. I had a lot of positive support and my friends would invite us all, including my father.

QUESTION: Were you given adequate information about the progression of the disease at the outset?

ANSWER: Yes. My therapist told us what to expect and we were forewarned. The doctors didn't tell me anything, because my father didn't visit doctors often and we took care of him at home.

QUESTION: What advice would you give the child of an Alzheimer patient at the outset of the disease? Near the end?

ANSWER: At the outset, I would suggest you get a good psychotherapist, someone you can trust and talk to. My therapist had a parent with the disease, too. Accept the fact that there is nothing you can do to make them well. It's just a matter of time.

QUESTION: What financial advice would you give?

ANSWER: Once your parents reach sixty to sixty-five, get everything out of their names, or you will lose everything.

▷ Laura is over sixty. She has one sister, one brother, and a husband who has been "marvelous." Her mother, diagnosed with dementia, is now ninety-four years old. Until her late eighties, her main problem was arthritis and being stuck in the house after her husband's death. She has deteriorated a lot in the last four years, and recognizes Laura only occasionally. Sometimes she's calm and sometimes she is "off the wall." Laura says she doesn't want to know "what she is" when she isn't visiting her.

QUESTION: What is the hardest part of seeing your mother go through the changes involved in her dementia?

ANSWER: The change in her appearance and the way she's dressed. She used to go to the beauty parlor every week. She had a lot of clothes, and was very meticulous in her appearance until her hands started shaking and she had coffee stains on her blouses. She constantly yells that she wants to go home, and my interpretation is that she wants to die.

QUESTION: Is there a role reversal? How do you feel about it?

ANSWER: Sure, there is: I feed her. It's my job! I try to feed her the ice cream that they give on Saturdays. I don't know what goes on a lot, because I can't deal with it.

QUESTION: Are you often angry or sad?
ANSWER: I don't feel angry, just helpless, knowing there's nothing I can do to make her more comfortable. There are even people worse than she is in there. She yells she wants to go home. We used to take her out in a wheelchair, but she always wanted to go back. Even inside, when we sat in the small lounge, she would want to go back to her room.

There used to be family members of patients that supported each other and took care of other patients, but they have died off, and now we are the old-timers. It was a family atmosphere then. It made it more palatable for us.

Am I often sad? Oh, yeah. To handle it, I just turn my mind off, and that bothers me. I have to, though; I have to go on with my life.

QUESTION: How do others around you relate to the patient and to you?
ANSWER: They all ask about her. The family members don't bother to come see her, except one cousin from out-of-state, and my mother's sister. I don't question, I don't want to make them feel guilty. They get upset when they see her.

My sister used to come more often, but now she can't. Sometimes my brother goes. My brother now works farther away, so he can't come on his way home until late, and by then my mother is very tired and totally nonfunctional.

QUESTION: Were you given adequate information about the progression of the disease at the outset?
ANSWER: No, not at all. Nobody even discussed it at the time. I just watched her degeneration. The shock was the way she reacted to the anesthesia in the hospital when she broke her hip. Would it have helped if I had been given more information? No, because I knew this was a natural progression of the disease.

About the health care workers in the nursing home: There is one very nice aide who has been there all along. (But there's supposed to be no tipping, and I really feel that I shouldn't tip her.) However, there is a very big turnover, otherwise. The charge nurse in charge of medication changes constantly. The members of the staff all come into my mother's room and know her name. But the administrator is very remote. The social worker is marvelous, and has been there since before my mother came. But she's part-time and overworked.

QUESTION: What mistakes have you made?
ANSWER: I wonder whether we could have put her into a home that had better facilities, with more occupational therapy. But we chose this place because it was convenient and it followed the dietary laws my mother cared about.

Also, my mother had a knee replacement operation ten years ago and never did the therapy then because it was painful. Since there was nobody in the house to push her, she didn't do it. Maybe I should have pushed her. But, on the other hand, the nursing home staff doesn't really want the residents to be mobile and slip on the floor. They prefer them in a wheelchair.

QUESTION: What advice would you give the child of a parent who was recently diagnosed with dementia?
ANSWER: It is not the child's fault, and both the parent and the child have no control over the situation.

QUESTION: What financial advice would you like to give?
ANSWER: As soon as someone retires, pay for a financial advisor—don't go to your cousin or your friend—and get good, sound advice. We got good advice after my mother had her knee operation. I just wish people could really put their finances in a proper state before there's trouble. Everyone should investigate long-term health care.

▷ Amy is over thirty. Her mother, past fifty, was officially diagnosed
  with Alzheimer's disease seven years before the interview. However, there were signs three or four years before that. She had been
  a teacher, a take-charge lady who always assured Amy that
  everything was going to be okay. Although Amy has a degree in
  guidance and counseling, she found that this experience was "a
  whole different ball game."

QUESTION: What is the hardest part of seeing your mother go
through the changes involved in Alzheimer's?
ANSWER: She's there but she's not; it's her body, but she is missing, lost inside in her own world, and I can't always reach her. Sometimes we hug or kiss, so if I close my eyes I can pretend it is the
way it used to be.

QUESTION: Is there a role reversal? How do you feel about it?
ANSWER: There definitely is a role reversal: I sit there feeding her
when I visit. Sometimes I do it jokingly, as I imagine she would have
fed me as a child. But she eats without any expression, so I tell her,
"Remember when you fed me?" and she doesn't respond. Sometimes she feeds herself, but it happens less and less as time goes on.

I sit with her while she is on the toilet, looking up at me. It
reminds me of all the times I used to be sitting on the toilet and
she was with me. I don't know what her level of comprehension
is, but if someone asks her for a kiss, she gives it. I don't think she
knows who I am. It's bizarre; there is no way to describe the feeling. It's the world standing on its end.

QUESTION: Are you often angry? What about sadness?
ANSWER: I was angry at her in the beginning, even though she used
to do little things to hide her condition and then pretend she was
playing a game. I didn't even want to see her right after the diagnosis. I couldn't even hug her. What changed it? Acceptance. The
early stages are a bigger nightmare than the deterioration that
follows, because you accept more as time passes. Acceptance
allowed me to be in the here and now, where she is.

There are tons of sadness. I couldn't talk about the disease until I had been in therapy for two years. It took a long time to work things out because I had to go through a lot of other stuff first, including my own chronic illness.

My feeling of being out of control was pure horror, out of the worst horror movie possible. I thought about how she used to brush her teeth and comb her hair and look the way she wanted. I wondered, if she ends up in a nursing home, who is going to dress her the way she likes? Of course, I didn't realize then that later on, you only want her clean. Now she just wears house dresses. I worry about the deterioration in hygiene. Her teeth could fall out, and then what? All this goes beyond the feelings of missing the person she used to be.

QUESTION: How do others around you relate to your mother and to you?
ANSWER: My husband is very supportive and good with her. She flirts with him. He holds her and kisses her, and that's a lot, because he married into this. He didn't get to meet her at her best. When he met her she already wasn't really herself.

People always ask about her and how she's doing, even though the answer will not be good. I'm pretty forward and frank about it: either it sucks or it doesn't. Sometimes I say, "Don't ask." They don't just brush it aside as though it wasn't a part of my life.

QUESTION: Were you given adequate information about the progression of the disease at the outset? How were the health care professionals you dealt with?
ANSWER: I went to the Alzheimer's organization and attended group meetings. In the groups, everything I was hearing dealt with the horrors of what was coming. I couldn't deal with what was, let alone with what was going to be, so I left the group. I learned little by little. It was so painful.

My mother was in an experimental drug program. The woman in charge of the program met with my mother regularly. Then she met with me. She recommended a therapist I could talk to one-on-one.

QUESTION: What are you most proud of?

ANSWER: I'm proud of my father. I see that the characteristics I didn't like before have carried him through this experience. His stubbornness served him and my mother quite well. He hasn't given up.

I'm totally grateful to him because I feel that he gave me life twice: first when I was born, and then when I married late and moved a hundred miles away with my husband. He gave us his blessings, giving me a guiltless second chance at life. That life is separate from him and my mother. That is why I do everything I can to be there for them.

QUESTION: Does going to your volunteer job help?

ANSWER: It fulfills another part of my needs in life, but it doesn't help me to deal with what is going on in my parents' life. I would still want to be doing that work if they were both in perfect health.

QUESTION: What mistakes have you made?

ANSWER: Just human mistakes, like not being more understanding and not being more loving. There were times when I stayed away from her, when she still knew who I was, because I was so angry at her for getting sick.

QUESTION: What advice would you give the child of a parent who was recently diagnosed with Alzheimer's?

ANSWER: The only thing that I can offer is not really advice. But I would like to tell this child that it is always going to hurt like hell, but the texture of the pain is going to change over time, and somehow you will make it through.

QUESTION: What financial advice would you like to give?

ANSWER: Go see an elder care lawyer ASAP. If you don't advocate for yourself and your family, you are asking for trouble. You must get the right information, as difficult as it is to hear or even to accept. There is a lot of avoidance, but everyone should get their financial house in order before the worst-case scenario hits.

> ▷ Mona Eve is a recent retiree whose mother lives in an out-of-state nursing home. She was diagnosed with Alzheimer's four years ago and has been in the home for six months. Mona Eve visits her mother approximately once a month, staying seven to fourteen days. One of her sisters supervises the mother's care. In spite of the distance, Mona Eve feels constantly burdened with concerns about her mother's welfare. There is a third sister who can't deal with their mother's illness or her care.

QUESTION: What is the hardest part of seeing your mother go through the changes involved in Alzheimer's?

ANSWER: To see a person who is no longer who she was, and then to see her intellectual and social awareness is diminishing and continues to diminish. And I can't share my life with her.

It was difficult to juggle my work schedule to go to see her, and I needed the job.

She was on medication at the beginning, but we found in a few months it wasn't doing any good, and it affected the liver as a side effect. They're coming out with new medications, but it will be too late for my mother. She's in pain with compression of some vertebrae and some residual bone damage from an old cancer that is recurring. X-rays didn't show it, but a bone scan did. She has poor circulation, angina, and cancer, and she's eighty-nine years old. Whatever goes, goes.

QUESTION: Is there a role reversal?

ANSWER: Not really. There was in the beginning, when she was throwing out money and gift certificates and I was dictating to her. But then I found out that is not the thing to do. She should be handled with give and take. Her rights and privileges, duties and responsibilities have to be considered. She was not formally diagnosed at first, we just thought senility was setting in.

QUESTION: Are you often angry? At what?

ANSWER: Not anymore. When she was at home and soiled the carpets because she didn't make it to the bathroom on time, I wasn't understanding or sympathetic. I prayed to learn patience. She would stand there in the middle of it and say, "I didn't do that. I don't know who did it, but it wasn't me." Once I saw how upset she was with herself, I developed more patience and understanding.

In the beginning, I would get angry over her situation, but I was able to reflect on it. I asked myself questions to understand what the emotion was, and then I was able to control it. Then the anger subsided.

QUESTION: How do you handle sadness?

ANSWER: I feel a whole gamut of emotions. I feel sad for her and I'm not sure I feel sad for myself. That is not a way to end your life, to not be cognizant of reality, to not know your children and grandchildren who have interesting lives. When I have some joy or sadness in my life I can't call her up and talk about it. I can't call her up about a medical problem for which she always used to have a tonic. She can't understand my words today; she thinks I'm saying another word. That makes it so unpleasant.

QUESTION: How do others around you relate to the patient and to you?

ANSWER: All the Alzheimer's people in her nursing home are on one floor with staff that has been specially trained, so they do well with her since they are used to it. Our family members also do well in her presence; they seem to be handling it. As for internally, I don't know.

I think most people don't understand what the disease is. The general public doesn't know. I think that's normal. Look at AIDS: people shut it out when it isn't in their lives. I would like to see more awareness of the disease. I would like people at the nursing home to ask for an autopsy of the brain to make further studies.

QUESTION: Were you given adequate information about the progression of the disease at the outset? How were the health care professionals you dealt with?

ANSWER: No, I wasn't given adequate information. That was gleaned from reading books. It would have helped if the health professionals had told me more. I want to know everything and have all the information. I did my own research, reading in the library and talking to people.

Even four years ago, people kept the disease kind of quiet, thinking there might be a stigma attached to it. It's the way that people used to shy away from even saying the word "cancer."

The doctor we dealt with the most was excellent, and he had a nice personality. He would come out to the waiting room to get her and make conversation with her. At that time she would banter back. We would rehearse before her visit, but she wouldn't remember, and she didn't know where she was or who the president was. She would answer by saying, "You work here, don't you know what building we're in?" She had great humor that could diffuse a situation. We thought that would continue.

The change didn't happen overnight, but it happened after she was in the home, where she was very unhappy at the beginning. It would be ideal to be able to keep someone at home, with twenty-four hours of caretaking in three eight-hour shifts. The caretakers need their quarters. You need a very big home and you need to afford that.

QUESTION: What are you most proud of?

ANSWER: I don't feel I'm in a position of pride at the moment. The person you once saw as the matriarch isn't the matriarch now. The image is fractured, even though I'm proud of the life she used to live. She believed in quality of life. The contrast is surreal. I feel my family has been taken away from me.

QUESTION: What mistakes have you made?

ANSWER: In the beginning, it was not understanding that you don't lecture or scold the person with dementia any more than you scold anyone in your family. It was her money she was throwing out the window. I didn't know that I couldn't have an open discussion with my mother.

QUESTION: Did going to work help?
ANSWER: It wasn't easier to be working. I used to spend a little less time with my mother, but today time away exceeds five days. I find packing once a month and going there to be a great interruption of my life. You're so far behind when you come back.

QUESTION: What advice would you give the child of a parent who was recently diagnosed with Alzheimer's?
ANSWER: Get involved with a support group. I personally don't think I could glean that much from a group. But for someone who was the primary caretaker, it would help, if it was a professionally run group. People have to find their own way, and what works for one doesn't work for another.

QUESTION: What financial advice would you like to give?
ANSWER: One doesn't know if someone is going to be diagnosed with this problem. The ill person's investments will just be eaten up.

I don't approve of people hiding their parents' money. We all can't fall on the state to support us. I think it's unfair to circumvent your responsibility because the next generation wants to get the money. The nursing home started at $4,000 a month and now has gone up for new admissions. You need some money to get into a good home. We could have chosen a cheaper home, but the money that she had goes for her.

I'm an advocate for long-term-care insurance.

▷ These interviews show that there are a variety of challenges the child of an Alzheimer's/dementia patient must overcome. There are also an unlimited number of ways of facing and dealing with the problems. It is possible to read, and read into, these interviews. So the next time you have trouble accepting your parent's forgetfulness and limitations, maybe referring to these accounts will help you to gain perspective. When you see your parent's disconnected actions and that makes you feel disconnected in turn, knowing others have survived these very traumas might give you comfort.

When you meet up with misery, you also meet wonderful people along the way. It is therefore hoped that you will gain strength and courage from these personal outpourings of caring children.

CHECKLIST

- ❏ Be prepared to deal with a variety of unexpected emotions, including anger at the person with dementia, sadness, and confusion.
- ❏ Work at reminding yourself that your parent has no control over what is happening. He/she is suffering from a disease of the brain.
- ❏ Explore your feelings about taking on the parental role as your parent becomes more childlike.
- ❏ Read up on the disease.
- ❏ Consider support groups appropriate for the child of a patient rather than the spouse.
- ❏ Clear up old misunderstandings while there is still time.
- ❏ Do what you can, but don't shoulder the entire responsibility by yourself. Hire someone if need be.
- ❏ Understand that some of your friends and family members will be unable to handle the situation.
- ❏ Maintain at least one of your favorite activities.
- ❏ See an elder law attorney right away, before your parent is paranoid or incompetent.

ADDITIONAL READING
ABOUT PARENTS WITH DEMENTIA

Hinnefeld, Joyce. *Everything You Need to Know When Someone You Love Has Alzheimer's Disease.* New York: Rosen Publishing Group, 1994.

McAndrews, Lynn. *My Father Forgets.* Maple City, Mich.: Northern Publishing, 1990.

Wilkinson, Beth. *Coping When a Grandparent Has Alzheimer's Disease.* New York: Rosen Publishing Group, 1992.

CHAPTER 10

A Year after Widowhood

Can it be that you survived a whole year? What a long and full year it seemed to be, too. You've done and felt more than you thought possible, right? You've explored new horizons. You've started on the new chapter in your life. A year isn't really that long a period of time. Don't feel that you must have finished everything you set out to do, or that you should even have a definite plan of action. However, now is a good time to look back and prepare to look forward.

First of all, have you taken care of the legal and financial odds and ends? If not, now is the time to attend to that. Consult a lawyer, a financial advisor, your accountant, or trusted friends to be sure you haven't overlooked anything. Check with the unclaimed funds department of your state. There may be some money you weren't aware of sitting out there. There is usually no fee involved: you just call up that division of the state tax department, and they kindly and clearly help you. They usually have a toll-free number.

Assess your financial situation. Will you be able to continue in your present lifestyle without making changes? Have you allowed for inflation, as well as for the fact that you may need more physical assistance in the future?

If cleaning the house isn't therapeutic, get someone else to do it for you, as a start. Ask around or call a college placement office to get help for yard work or clerical work. If you can't afford to spend the money, work out an exchange deal with someone you know: both of you will help each other with paperwork, or one will handle some chore in exchange for some other. Be creative, and reach out. No one can guess that you need help unless you tell them. In any case, having an appointment to do something with someone else will guarantee that you'll work on it. It will also make the job easier and more than twice as fast as doing it alone. As a result, even if you give the other person an amount of time equal to what he/she gives you, you're ahead of the game.

A very important and difficult task is giving away the clothes of the deceased. It's something I could not have done alone. I hired a teenager. She was tolerant of my tears and reminiscences. I volunteered to help someone in my bereavement group to go through her husband's things in exchange for her cooking me some meals. If a certain item holds too much meaning for you to give it up, keep it. Eventually, you'll either use it as a soothing souvenir, or you'll discard it.

What to do with the clothes? It is often easier to give things to someone we know who can use them. But there are bound to be articles of clothing no one you know wants to "adopt." You can give them to charity. Make sure they are clean and presentable. Make a list of all the items and what you think they are worth used. (If you have no idea of how to evaluate your donations, go to a thrift shop to get an idea of prices.) Deliver the clothes, and other things for that matter, to a charity of your choice or have them picked up by appointment. Your phone book has a list of local charities. I would not suggest leaving things on a porch for pickup since I once had a few such bags disappear without a trace. The charity left a message on my answering machine asking why I hadn't put them out.

Speaking of answering machines, if you don't have one, if you don't like them, if you are afraid of them, consider getting one anyway. Sure, the callers can always call back. But you are at a time in your life when you will feel better knowing that someone did call. You don't want to miss any important information, financial or other. Also, unless you only have brief telephone conversations, do yourself and your callers the favor of getting call waiting. You don't have to be rude about asking someone to please hold on for a moment, and you can return the call later on. The advantages are guilt-free long conversations and sparing your friends the frustration of trying to get through. Of course, you could also get a second phone line!

When you donate clothing and other useful articles to charity, you not only help those who can't afford to buy new, but you also earn yourself a tax deduction. If the value of your donation is more than $250, you will have show how and where you obtained these things: were they gifts or purchases? Although that's no big deal, if you want to avoid another clerical chore at tax time, make donations under this amount.

Now that the dust has settled, so to speak, it's time for you to prepare your own estate plan (see chapter 6). Take a look at your old will. Does it still do what you want it to? How about giving some things or money away now so you can see the ones you care about enjoy them? Or, of course, spend more. One saying that keeps changing its implications is "You should die poor." How about interpreting that to mean that you shouldn't hesitate to spend money for what you need or want? It's not wise to spend it recklessly, but why not allow yourself to leave a little less to your heirs, and make your life easier and more enjoyable? If you don't use your money to enjoy yourself, you can bet your children (or others) will use it to enjoy *themselves!*

A lot of people will want to give you financial advice, often with a commission attached. Read up on what you don't know (see the list at the end of this chapter), browse in the financial advice section of your local library, and listen to radio financial talk shows. Keep your checkbook closed. Never give any money to anyone who calls you out of the blue. Insist that everything be in writing. Remember, if it seems too good to be true, it is. If the deal is so hot it can't wait, it will burn you, guaranteed. You will be the poorer for it. You will also feel foolish and embarrassed.

Generally speaking, the greater the income from an investment, the greater the risk. You might not make a killing on the stock market by investing in government bonds, but you won't lose any of your principal, either. Put your money into whatever lets you sleep at night. As you educate yourself about a variety of possible investments, you will be able to make intelligent decisions. Then, if you want to gamble on futures or sit tight with a well-established blue-chip stock, you'll do it with assurance.

Not all the people approaching you about money will be strangers. Your children may have some ideas, too. Resist the temptation to do what they suggest just because you don't want to lose their love. If that's all their love rests on, you can bet that you'll lose it anyway. Most children want what's best for their parents. If they come up with an idea that helps them as well, it's probably well-meant. But, for example, if you don't really want to sell your home and move into a house with them, don't.

If you don't want to move in with a child, but want to give him/her your house, think it through. If you put the deed to your house in a child's name, consider the emotional and financial consequences: are there any other children who would feel left out? If one child is more successful, does he/she agree that you should give the homestead to a sibling? In addition, if the home is no longer in your name, you are a tenant in someone else's house. You could be evicted. That's rare, but it happens more often than you'd think. What happens even more often is divorce. Would you want your home involved in a divorce settlement?

Giving your child or children the house may not save them as much money and hassle as you think. When you give your house to someone, the cost basis (the purchase price plus the cost of improvements) remains what it was when you first bought the house. When someone inherits a property, the cost basis is its value on the date of your death. So when your house is sold, the profit (called capital gain) is greater and the tax consequences are greater if you've given the house away before your death. Such a gift also requires your filing gift tax forms and dealing with a competent accountant. There are no federal taxes on inheritances up to $675,000, and that exemption will grow annually to a cap of $1 million in the year 2006. If you have more money than that, you should be doing some extra planning, anyway. Although many states tax smaller inheritances than the IRS, the percentage of their cut is lower than the federal percentages.

If you own a house, and it's your main asset, you might also want to hold on to it for a reverse mortgage, which you might need if you live to a ripe old age and are short of cash. Reverse mortgages are becoming more common. Here's how they work: Whatever cash value your house has can be used as collateral to get a bank loan, either in monthly payments, as a lump-sum payout, or in a line of credit. When you move (or move on), the house is sold and the bank is paid back whatever it lent you, plus a percentage of the principal for interest, of course. A reverse mortgage can be a good solution for an older person who is house-rich and cash-poor but doesn't want to sell the house.

Before you sign up with any lender, compare plans using the total annual loan costs. Those can include interest, closing costs, origination fees, points, mortgage insurance, and servicing fees. If your reverse mortgage agreement includes an annuity, make sure you understand the cost of that, too.

If you have substantial assets and would like to give some to your favorite charity, consider a charitable remainder trust. There are a variety of them, but I'll outline the basic idea here: You donate an asset, preferably one that has appreciated in value, since the charity won't have to pay any capital gains taxes, and you will be granted a charitable tax deduction for the current value of the asset. The IRS evaluates the donation according to certain charts, which means that you will not be credited dollar for dollar. But it's a good deal anyway since this donation entitles you to a large tax credit, and often a big refund. With that refund, you can buy a single-premium life insurance policy worth more upon your death than the asset you have just donated, so your heirs lose nothing, and may even gain more. You could also invest the refund in any financial vehicle of your choosing.

Once such a trust is set up, the charity will give you a yearly distribution of a pre-agreed amount of money. Sounds great, right? Unfortunately, this can't be done by just any lawyer or accountant. You must check carefully with the charity and with the IRS to be sure this procedure is done correctly by the right professionals.

You may have a completely different situation: you may be in a rented apartment and be struggling financially. Remember, Social Security offers widow/er's benefits, as well as SSI, Supplemental Security Income. You might be entitled to food stamps. You do not necessarily have to wait for hours in long lines. First, call Social Security at (800) 772-1213. Then, look in the phone book for agencies for the elderly (also look in the resources section). The staff at agencies for the aging can give you information and assistance if you are short of funds. It takes time and patience, and often perseverance, but you can get help. If someone doesn't call you back, you call again. The agencies are often understaffed and overworked. You know, the squeaky wheel gets the grease. But a little sugar helps too; being unpleasant won't get you as far.

Should you turn to your children for help or advice? That depends on the relationship that you have with them, of course, but by and large, a trusted outsider can be more impartial and less emotionally involved. You might not want to upset your children or have them upset you. If you've never had a talk about finances before, go slowly and carefully, and pick a neutral location to start the discussion.

Speaking of children, you probably have found some comfort in the role reversal that took place when you were first bereaved, and the younger generation sort of took over some of your responsibilities. Now is the time to thank them, treat them to something special as a thank-you, and start taking charge of your own affairs again. You might feel shaky at first, but soon enough, you will enjoy the independence and freedom. It's nice to be able to give yourself a pat on the back and to realize that you are ready to move on.

Moving on doesn't require that you give up your memories. Nor does it mean that the pain will suddenly go away. It's still there, in the back of your head, at the base of your neck. But somehow it becomes enveloped in layers of insulation brought on by day-to-day living and new experiences, so it hurts less with time. The day actually comes when that lump of sadness is not the first thing you become aware of when you wake up.

When you want to feel close to the deceased, you can still find comfort in going to visit the grave of your loved one, if that's possible. Although you will probably find yourself talking to him/her often wherever you are, at the gravesite the communication seems more real, more intimate. You can touch the stone, feel the outline of the lettering. Those extra physical contacts are a solace, and the better you feel emotionally, the better you will feel physically.

To feel less lonely, you may want to get a pet, if you don't already have one. Studies have shown that the presence of an animal in your life brings consolation and a feeling of worth. The owner needs this companion as much as he/she is needed by the animal. Pets are always near, long after people have gone about their business and forgotten the recently bereaved. Besides, a furry creature is a great source of hugs and petting, which relax you and lower your blood pressure. It is in times of loneliness that one is more susceptible to illness, and anything that helps maintain health is an advantage.

That brings up health insurance. You probably had your fill of paperwork when you were an active caregiver, but it is important to verify that you have the health coverage that you need. If you are on Medicare, Part B will cover 80 percent of your out-of-hospital medical bills, after a yearly deductible, if you use participating doctors. A great many physicians participate. You should consider some type of "medigap" policy to cover the other 20 percent. Be careful, though, that you don't pay for unnecessary duplicate coverage. Also make sure that the secondary insurance will pay in addition to the Medicare payment, not instead of it. Please keep in mind that secondary insurance will only pay if Medicare approves the expense. Since details of Medicare coverage are constantly changing, it would be wise for you to call Medicare or a senior agency for advice.

As for Medicare Part A, it covers hospital stays completely, except for a deductible, for a period of sixty days in a row. For days sixty-one through ninety, you must pay a daily co-payment. If you're discharged before the first sixty days are up, and then are readmitted within another sixty days, the clock resumes ticking on the allotment from the previous stay. If you're out of the hospital at least sixty days in a row, and then go back in, another sixty-day period of full coverage begins, with another deductible, and another thirty days of coverage with co-payment. If you should end up having to stay in a hospital for longer than ninety days (sixty days of full coverage plus thirty days of coverage with a daily co-payment), you can dip into your one-time lifetime reserve of sixty days. Medicare will cover all expenses except for another daily co-payment amount. If you use any of these reserve days, you must sign papers to the effect that you realize that you are taking days from your lifetime reserve fund. For further information, contact Medicare at (800) 633-4227. Their operators are quite patient and gentle. You can also get details of Medicare coverage at http://www.medicare.gov. If you don't have a computer, a local library or senior center should have access to this Web site.

All the Part A benefits are free coverage. You must pay monthly premiums for Part B, though. That's why HMOs seem attractive to seniors who want to save on the monthly premiums. Think very, very carefully before you give up your Medicare coverage because some other organization promises you something better. Read and understand everything you sign. You don't want any nasty surprises at the time of an illness, when you are the most vulnerable.

If you're not eligible for Medicare, see what your employer or former employer can offer. You can buy private health insurance, but it's quite expensive. At the very least, buy hospitalization coverage. It's in a hospital that the charges really add up. Look into the offerings of organizations for seniors like AARP or private societies you are eligible to join. To leave yourself without any protection is foolhardy, unless, of course, you have no assets to speak of and will be immediately eligible for Medicaid. In that case, you can go

to see doctors in free clinics, and your hospital stays in certain facilities will be covered. You need a lot of patience and a good book
to read or project to work on when you go because the wait is
shamefully long in many clinics. But they do attend to your needs.
If you're uncomfortable with the doctor you have seen, don't hesitate to ask to see another one at a later date.

Besides health insurance, do you need long-term-care insurance?
That depends on what assets you need to protect and on how
high a premium you can afford to pay. Even if you decide you need
the insurance, you may have trouble getting accepted for a policy.
People over fifty and in good health are often turned down. Medicare doesn't generally pay for an unlimited nursing home stay. It
pays completely for the first twenty days in a skilled nursing facility if you were transferred directly from a hospital to which you
were admitted for medical reasons. For the next eighty days, it pays
for all covered services except for a daily co-payment. That amount
of time is usually adequate to recuperate from a broken hip and
go home to be on your own, but all sorts of other things can happen. That's why it pays, in peace of mind as well as in dollars, to
buy medigap and long-term-care insurance. Contact major insur-
ers, ask your doctor's secretary, and gather as much information
for comparison as you can before you sign up for any coverage.

Although Medicare will not pay for what they call "custodial
care" when that's the only kind of care you need (help in getting
dressed, bathing, or eating), it will pay the full cost of home health
visits from one of their approved agencies if you are confined to
your home and have a medical condition that warrants the regular visit of a nurse. The number of visits you might be entitled to
is unlimited.

As you can see, there are many aspects to medical coverage. The
suggested reading list at the end of this chapter will enable you to
explore more possibilities, and I urge you to do some extra reading on the matter. Also see chapter 6 on Medicaid eligibility. The
point is, you must decide how to handle the future health problems that might come up.

While you're making such decisions, you should also consider your end-of-life choices: prepare a living will, which is not a legal document, but a guide for those who might have to make crucial decisions about your medical treatments if you are unable to do so. A health care proxy is a legal document, but it is not available or valid in all states—something to keep in mind when you are traveling. You can contact an organization like Partnership for Caring for details (also see the resources section). If you do not want to have life supports, including a stomach tube or artificial hydration, you must put your wishes in writing. Give a copy of your directives to your physician as well as to the individuals you will count on to enforce your wishes. A word of caution: the person you feel closest to will not necessarily obey your wishes. Not everyone can resist prolonging someone's life or can disregard the suggestions of medical personnel who may want to keep a patient alive as long as possible.

If, on the other hand, you do want to stay on this earth as long as medical science can enable you to, you must also specify that, so your loved ones will be empowered to order the necessary treatments making that possible.

The last in a list of insurances is life insurance. Do you need any? Is there anyone you have to protect in case of your death? If there isn't, save on the premiums and invest in something else. Keep in mind, however, that if your estate will generate large inheritance taxes, a life insurance policy will make it much easier on your heirs. First of all, taxes are due early on, possibly before the estate is settled. Secondly, you might not want the inheritance to be reduced by the amount of taxes. Most people know that life insurance money goes directly to the beneficiary without having to go through probate, but many don't know that the value of the policy counts as part of the estate. The best way to avoid that is to have the beneficiaries own the policy on your life. If you don't want them to pay the yearly premiums, gift them the amount of the premium when the bill comes. Remember that you can give anyone ten thousand dollars a year tax-free for as many years as you want.

Now that all those technicalities are out of the way, you can relax and develop your social life. Not everyone wants to find a new partner. If they do want to find one, these days they don't necessarily want to get married. They don't want to have the responsibilities they had before. The fact of the matter is, though, if you love someone, whether you're married or not, you'll be affected by that person's illness. Also, if you are the sweetheart instead of the spouse, the person's children have control over what happens to him/her, and might even exclude you completely. On the other hand, a prenuptial agreement will protect you in case of divorce or death, but carries no weight with Medicaid, since both spouses' money is eligible to be used for treatment and care of either spouse.

If you have decided that romance is not for you, you will draw upon your circle of friends and family to entertain and surround you at special occasions. You will probably meet new friends as time goes on and you participate in various activities, but you most likely won't be searching for a lot of additional friends. Such is not the case if you want a sweetheart. Should you seek another companion, you can locate information on the topic by reading local papers, going to the library, or visiting the Internet.

No matter what your social life may be, you're on the go. The future is open to you. You may bump into disappointments, in the dating world or elsewhere. You know you've picked yourself up and dusted yourself off before. You can do it again. Whatever path you take, may your curiosity be aroused about a dozen things, and may you enjoy exploring at least half of them. It might sound corny, but there's always tomorrow. That's when you will be able to do what you want, when you want, and how you want to do it.

CHECKLIST

- ❑ Attend to all unfinished legal and financial business.
- ❑ Decide on what lifestyle you want, keeping your financial and physical limitations in mind.
- ❑ Verify that you have cleared out all unnecessary clothes and personal belongings of your loved one.

❑ Look into your own estate plan and your insurance needs (life insurance, long-term-care insurance, health care, and hospitalization). Make out a living will and/or health care proxy.

❑ Educate yourself about investments. Until you do, park your funds in a very safe, conservative investment that is government insured. Study up on reverse mortgages, should you ever need one.

❑ Decide what you want from your children or other relatives, what you want to give them in time and money, and talk to them about it all.

❑ Consider the advantages of charitable giving, with the help of a knowledgeable professional.

❑ If you need financial aid, find out what is out there by contacting Social Security and senior agencies.

❑ Choose the type of socializing you would be most comfortable with and, if appropriate, look for announcements of singles events in the newspaper. Tell those around you you're ready to date, if you are. Try the personal ads.

❑ Evaluate your outlook on sex and act accordingly.

❑ Buy an answering machine if you don't have one, and sign up for call waiting if possible.

ADDITIONAL READING ABOUT MOVING ON

Berg, Adriane G. *Warning: Dying May Be Hazardous to Your Wealth.* Franklin Lakes, N.J.: Career Press, 1992.

Browne, Joy. *Dating for Dummies.* Foster City, Calif.: IDG Books, 1997.

Canfield, Jack, et al. *Chicken Soup for the Surviving Soul.* Deerfield Beach, Fla.: Health Communications, 1996.

Carlson, Richard. *Don't Sweat the Small Stuff, and It's All Small Stuff.* New York: Hyperion, 1997.

Englander, Debra Wishik. *Money 101.* Rocklin, Calif.: Prima Publishing, 1997.

Epstein, Alan. *How to Be Happier Day by Day—A Year of Mindful Actions.* New York: Penguin Books, 1993.

Fensterheim, Herbert, and Jean Baer. *Don't Say Yes When You Want to Say No.* New York: Dell, 1998.

Finley, Guy. *The Secret of Letting Go.* St. Paul, Minn.: Llewellyn Publications, 1997.

Fulghum, Robert. *From Beginning to End: The Rituals of Our Lives.* New York: Ivy Books, 1995.

Guide to Health Insurance for People with Medicare. Health Care Financing Administration of the U.S. Department of Health and Human Services, (800) 638-6833.

Inlander, Charles B., and Michael A. Donio. *Medicare Made Easy.* Allentown, Pa.: People's Medical Society, 1999.

Medicare and You 2000. Baltimore, Md.: Federal Medicare Agency of the Health Care Financing Administration.

Partnership for Caring publications. 1035 30th Street NW, Washington, D.C. 20007.

Wiegold, C. Frederic, ed. *The Wall Street Journal Lifetime Guide to Money.* New York: Hyperion, 1997.

CHAPTER 11

Comments Overheard at Support Group Meetings

When I attended Alzheimer's support group meetings, I was often struck by the wisdom of some of the things that were said spontaneously. These statements overheard at meetings give insight into the thoughts and feelings of caregivers. They also give advice in a subtle way. That's why I collected them and I'm including them here. I hope you find them enlightening.

▷ When dealing with other family members, it's easier to beg forgiveness than to ask permission.

▷ You just can't reason with him. You shouldn't even try.

▷ Life is so time-consuming!

▷ A friend eating with us at a restaurant said: "Look! He's eating his salad with a knife." I answered, "You tell him."

▷ A friend of mine called while I was out. He told her that I would be back "in a short distance."

▷ Be mad at the illness, not at the person.

▷ My mantra has become, "It's the disease talking."

▷ I remind myself that he has a short-circuit in the brain, but sometimes that doesn't help at that moment.

▷ I don't mind that he insists on dressing himself and then dresses totally inappropriately, but when he stands there turning the lights on and off nonstop, I want to scream.

▷ I love her. I want to help her. I empathize. But darn it, there are moments that are so frustrating that I think my burnout is going to come in a flash, and I'll just go up in a puff of smoke.

▷ Because my mother still looks like my mother, I feel frustrated because she doesn't behave like my mother.

▷ Even though there were stamps right there, on the desk, I answered his request that I go buy some stamps with, "You're right, I'll get you some stamps."

▷ When I was crying in front of my grown child, I said, "Just give me tissues and shut up."

▷ I have it together; I just don't remember where I put it.

▷ I'm so scared I'll get it, too.

▷ I started noticing a difference when I bought her a microwave oven. It was too complicated for her, and she got mad at me.

▷ He gave up his interest in everything. He had a complete personality reversal.

▷ He's lost all of his communicating skills.

▷ Looking back, I realize there were significant changes, but I just didn't realize what they meant at the time. Maybe it was better that way.

▷ When the checks started to bounce, I didn't get it. I thought he was just getting older, that's all.

▷ He couldn't total up a restaurant tab or figure out the tip.

▷ He couldn't make the connection between the fork, the food, and his mouth.

▷ Most people out there aren't aware of what we're going through.

▷ We're exhausted, confused, and need a pat on the back.

▷ We give the caring to the sick person. Who gives us the caring?

▷ A phone call is so precious.

▷ The whole world disappears.

▷ Friends and family don't understand, and they pull back.

▷ At least this group makes me feel less isolated, even if it's only for a short while.

▷ I feel safe here, and I can say anything, even if it sounds awful.

▷ When it reached a point where he ripped off his diapers and smeared the feces on the wall, I felt as though I was the victim.

▷ There's nothing to do except buy a supply of disinfectant and put linoleum on the floor.

▷ I know it will all be over one day, but I dread the emptiness.

▷ Selective memory helps. I try to remember the good times.

▷ Although she has trouble remembering recent events, the things that happened long ago are crystal clear in her mind.

▷ Now that she is less able to function, it's easier in a way.

▷ It used to rip my heart out when she would cry about losing her mind, not knowing or understanding what was happening.

▷ I couldn't handle the terror in her eyes.

▷ When we got him a hearing aid, he was less "out of it."

▷ This is the hardest job I've ever had. Thank goodness I'm doing it out of love. No amount of money could be enough.

▷ I've learned not to give her any choices. I don't tell her what we're *going* to do, I just tell her what to do directly, at that moment. It takes some thinking ahead, but it avoids a lot of conflicts.

▷ I'm so glad we can still hug.

▷ When we laugh together, it feels like old times. But when we cry, it's the present. Still, we're together in our emotions when we're sad. That means a lot to me.

▷ I'm so grateful we made financial decisions at the beginning. It would be too late now.

▷ The red tape I have to go through to get help is too much at times. But when all the paperwork and phone calls are done, I'm glad I arranged for whatever.

▷ She used to be so modest, and now, she doesn't care who sees her naked. At least that makes it easier to have my daughter help me give her a shower, but still . . .

▷ Once he got settled in the nursing home, I didn't feel so guilty. I sort of feel guilty about *that!*

▷ I cried and cried after I hit him. I promised myself I wouldn't ever do that again. Then I did it again, just a few days later. That's why he's better off in a nursing home. I'm better off, too.

▷ I can't believe the sun keeps rising every day.

▷ You gotta have faith. In what, I'm not sure, but you just gotta have faith.

CHAPTER 12

Frequently Asked Questions and Answers about Dementia

As I acquired more and more information and survival skills, other caregivers would ask me questions of all sorts. There were also questions that came up in the support group that had no ready answers at that moment. I found those answers while doing research for this book. I thought you might benefit from a list, since a lot of these questions are in the minds of many caregivers of people with dementia.

QUESTION: How do I know I'm not getting Alzheimer's, too?
ANSWER: Being forgetful does not by itself indicate Alzheimer's. Fatigue and stress can prevent you from thinking clearly. To play it safe, make an appointment with a neurologist to be checked out thoroughly. Your family physician also might be of help, but he/she doesn't usually have access to sophisticated testing equipment. He/she also may not have had as much experience with dementia as a neurologist. A psychiatrist also might be of help. It will be worth the time and money to get peace of mind.

QUESTION: How can I get help with laundry, cooking, and general housework without paying a fortune?

ANSWER: Contact your local government representative's office. The staff there should be able to guide you to the right senior resources. Once you speak to one person in one division, you will be referred to many others. You could also look in the phone book for listings of senior centers. Even though they don't supply such services, they should be able to give you good leads.

If you're able to pay for some help, contact the nearest church and tell the staff there what your needs are. Churches often know of people who need work and can put you in touch with someone. Then, there's always word-of-mouth, so ask around to see whether anyone has a lead.

Remember, though, that the least important thing to be concerned about now is how clean the house is. Dust can be removed at any time, and dirty floors never killed anyone. Food and laundry are crucial, so concentrate on them. (Don't worry about what people will say. Let them help you, or let them think what they will. Only someone who's "been there" really understands.)

QUESTION: Can I get Meals-on-Wheels if we're not on Medicaid?
ANSWER: Yes, you can. Although you yourself might not be eligible, the patient usually is. Call your local senior center for advice on how to sign up.

QUESTION: What about transportation? How can I get relief from all the chauffeuring I have to do?
ANSWER: First, see whether any friends might take your loved one to an occasional appointment. If anyone says, "Is there anything I can do to help?" take them up on it. If they don't want to do it again, you'll at least have had one moment of respite.

You can also contact your local senior center or government official to find out what your loved one is entitled to. You should mention that it will be necessary for you to accompany him/her, and find out what arrangements are available to allow that. Remember, you are not the only one in this kind of situation. There are solutions.

QUESTION: What happens when the money runs out? Should I exhaust all my savings?

ANSWER: You must keep a reserve of funds for yourself. Even the government allows you to have some money in the bank when you or your loved one become eligible for Medicaid (see chapter 6). Make necessary repairs on your home, prepay funeral arrangements, pay the year's real estate or other taxes, and spend some money on good, healthy food for the both of you. Then you can consider applying for Medicaid, which will entitle you to a good deal of help.

QUESTION: Just what does Medicare cover?

ANSWER: It will cover a percentage of medical necessities, but not custodial care. That means that it will pay for a certain amount of time in a nursing home if it is a medical necessity, but not if the patient needs help with daily activities like eating and bathing and has no other medical problem (again, see chapter 6).

QUESTION: How can I find the right doctor?

ANSWER: Ask for recommendations from friends, relatives, or support group members. If you have a doctor you like, even a specialist in an unrelated field, ask him/her for a recommendation. You can also call your local medical association. That means you won't have a personal recommendation, but maybe you'd rather not rely on someone else's opinion.

If you are meeting a physician for the first time, you might want to speak to him/her on the phone before your visit, or ask to speak to him/her alone at first, since you may want to talk about certain things out of earshot of your loved one.

Make a list of the things that concern you. If you don't have a list to look at, you'll probably forget to ask something that is important to you. Don't hesitate to ask questions, even if you think they're too basic. You need to know answers, and the doctor's attitude will help you to decide whether or not you want to return.

QUESTION: Where can I buy diapers and other products I use daily in bulk?

ANSWER: First, ask your local druggist. Then contact the company listed on the package of the product that you like. Another source is your local paper, where there may be an ad placed by someone who no longer needs the large supply he/she has. That would save you money, too. You could also look at the ads in senior magazines. They may give you productive leads for mail order. Take a look in your public library for a selection of magazines aimed at the elderly. Also, look at the resource lists at the end of this book.

I would encourage you to get a generous supply. If you buy items by the case, you might get a discount. If you mail order them, you don't have to do the carrying, and the cost might be advantageous. In any case, you don't want to be running low at the most inconvenient time.

QUESTION: Where can I write to complain about bad treatment my loved one is getting?

ANSWER: That depends on where the treatment is, but you should first start with an immediate superior. If your problem is with a doctor in private practice, you can find the address of the local medical society in your phone book. They will help you in filing a complaint. It is in their best interest to see to it that doctors in the area do not act out of line, and they do investigate. If someone you know suggests that you sue, remember that it's not so easy to go to court. It takes a lot out of you emotionally as well as financially. So, try the medical society route first, since that's actually easier, and certainly cheaper than starting a court case. There is still time to hire a lawyer later on, although there is a statute of limitations in most states.

If your problem is in a hospital, start with a floor supervisor and also contact the hospital patient ombudsman. If you get no satisfaction, go to the head of a department, and eventually, to the head of the hospital. If you still need satisfaction after that, and feel you have a good case, you can contact the federal Joint Commission on

Accreditation of Healthcare Organizations (see chapter 5). If they can't help you, they should be able to tell you who can. Unfortunately, though, thoughtless treatment or inconsiderate manners do not rate as major reasons for complaints. So, if the problem is not really major, take a deep breath and move on. Save your energy for bigger issues.

If you have a complaint about the treatment in a nursing home, there are also regulatory agencies to contact after you have gone up the ladder as outlined above. Look in the yellow pages under "Nursing Homes" and take it from there. Within a few phone calls, you'll have the information you need (again, see chapter 5).

Most of all, remember the expression "Vote with your feet" and look for another person or facility if things are really bad. Don't be shy. If you know what's good for the person you care about, and you know what's bad, it's perfectly OK to do something to correct an unsatisfactory situation.

QUESTION: How can I find a good lawyer?
ANSWER: Ask around or call your local bar association. There is a list of questions you can ask a potential elder law lawyer in chapter 6.

QUESTION: What can I do to feel less tired?
ANSWER: Eliminate anything that isn't really necessary or doesn't make you feel good. That includes contact with people who aren't supportive or who make you feel uncomfortable. You must consider your well-being. Listen to those who are helpful and ignore the others. Also, get an answering machine, return calls only when you really feel up to it, and keep the conversations short. Use a timer if need be. You can also get some stationery and write a quick note if a phone conversation doesn't suit you. You need sleep. You get precious little of it. If falling asleep is difficult, you can speak to your doctor about it. You can also try deep breathing, pleasant scents around your pillow, music, or distracting sounds that soothe you enough to enable you to fall asleep. I myself found that increasing

my calcium intake worked wonders, and I always went to sleep within two minutes. (Too bad the alarm always went off way too soon!)

QUESTION: How long will all this last?
ANSWER: There really is no way to tell. It all depends on the physical health of the patient. A duration of ten years is not unusual. That's why it's so important for you to maintain your own emotional and physical strength.

QUESTION: What do I do when she refuses to get off the toilet seat for hours?
ANSWER: If all attempts to move her fail, and you don't want to call 911 for emergency help, just wait it out. Give her food or drink as necessary, and let her doze off for a while. When she wakes up, you will most likely be able to matter-of-factly suggest that she go to bed, or wherever it is you want her to be at that point. You might want to read to her or listen to music together. It may not be the most glamorous spot, and may not be the greatest for her anatomy (yanking her would be more painful and useless if she resists), but you can turn an unpleasant incident to a sweet memory.

Try distracting her for a moment, and then guide her to another location. But if she's stubborn about it, shouting or threatening won't help. It's unlikely that you can pick her up (as you would a baby), so your options are limited. This is one case when you might have to come late or even cancel your appointment. However, don't stay at her side if she's being difficult. Be nearby, but read or write a letter, or do something you were going to do later on, anyway.

Just remember that this, too, shall pass. Maybe you can see the humor in it.

QUESTION: How can I control his tendency to roam?
ANSWER: Put locks high up or low down where he won't see them, or get a lock with a key for inside the door, and keep the key with you. Get an ID bracelet that specifies "memory impaired." If he's outside and doesn't want to come in, walk with him a moment,

then suggest that you both go home for a warm/cold drink, to eat, to get out of the cold, or whatever you think of on the spur of the moment.

It's important that you not get upset. It won't help. Threats or pleading are unlikely to work, since he can't reason enough to understand them. So just play along for a while, and you'll both be home soon enough.

To lessen nighttime wandering, you can try to reduce naps in the daytime, and have the patient do more physical exercise during the day, too. Why not take a daily walk together? Also, cover mirrors and remove distractions like bright objects, which could be disorienting in the middle of the night.

Put childproof gates at the top of stairs, have night lights, and generally make the house safe in case the person wanders while you are asleep.

QUESTION: What is "sundowning syndrome"?
ANSWER: It's the label given to explain why many people with dementing illnesses behave less well as the day comes to a close. To minimize the effects of this phenomenon, schedule complicated activities earlier in the day. Put off things like giving a shower if it's too stressful. Eliminate as many noises as you can. Dim some lights. Speak calmly and softly. Soothing music might help both of you.

QUESTION: How can I deal with the repetitive questions? She asks the same question ten to twenty times, one right after the other!
ANSWER: After you answer initially, try to ignore the question, unless she gets upset. If she can still read, make up index cards with the answers to questions she asks often. If she does get upset, just answer and try to be reassuring. The reason she keeps asking is that she can't process the information. On some level, that can be frustrating to her as well as to you. Try distracting her right after you answer the question. Play some music, sing a song, read a poem out loud. That will soothe you, besides.

QUESTION: How should I handle the insults and the complaints?

ANSWER: Don't argue or contradict, no matter how tempting that is. It will only agitate the person. Remember that what you are hearing is the disease talking, not the person you care about. If you're angry or upset yourself, go into another room for a few moments to compose yourself. Remind yourself what it is you're dealing with, and why it is you want to take care of this person. Take a breather, read, watch TV, or listen to music.

QUESTION: How can I stop him from going through my stuff and hiding things?

ANSWER: You can't stop him, you can only make it harder to do. Lock things up. Keep the house neat and uncluttered so he can find the things he's looking for. If your loved one is still able to be independent, make a list of where things are and hang it where it will be easy to see. That way, he won't have to rummage through so much to find what he's looking for.

QUESTION: He exposed himself! How can I prevent that from ever happening again?

ANSWER: You may not be able to. It is sometimes a part of the disease. Do your best not to react strongly, because that will only upset him and make him difficult to handle. Simply walk him to a private place. Then try distraction. If he's doing it at home, let it be, if it isn't too bothersome to you.

QUESTION: She follows me everywhere. How can I have some privacy?

ANSWER: Lead her to a limited, safe area. If she can still understand, set a timer and explain that you will return when the timer rings. Give her a task that she can do, like folding and unfolding towels, even if there's no need for the towels to be folded. Then, disappear behind a closed door. A few minutes alone will work wonders for you.

QUESTION: She has hallucinations. How do I handle that?

ANSWER: Remember that, to her, they're real. Reassure her. Don't challenge her, but don't agree with her, either. Stay neutral. Try distracting her as soon as she's calmer. If this happens often, discuss it with her doctor.

QUESTION: How can I deal with his suspicions and false accusations?

ANSWER: Keep in mind that he has no control over his thoughts. He may be feeling lost, confused, or distressed. Don't contradict him, just be sympathetic and reassuring. Then distract him in some way. If he is constantly paranoid, speak to the doctor about it. Anti-paranoia drugs may help.

QUESTION: How can I avoid his unexpected outbursts? Should I avoid all mental stimulation?

ANSWER: Everyday tasks may upset him even though they seem simple to you. Don't give him a task that requires him to think of more than one thing at a time. Try to identify with his frustration, and be as sensitive as you can. He does need some kind of mental stimulation, but it must be broken down to its simplest elements.

QUESTION: She does the same thing over and over, sometimes for hours. Is it OK for me to let her?

ANSWER: Sure, it's OK. She's not aware of the passage of time, and doing something, even again and again, makes her feel good. She doesn't realize that she's doing the same thing so many times. Take advantage of her being busy to accomplish something for yourself.

QUESTION: What medication is available?

ANSWER: Your neurologist is the one who is most likely to be up on the latest developments in the field. Unfortunately, there isn't any foolproof medication on the market as yet, although there are some products that will sometimes slow down the progress of the disease when they are administered at the onset of the dementia. There are others that will make a patient in an advanced stage less aggressive. Usually in cooperation with a doctor, you will have to try out a number of things to find something that works. Unfortunately, what works at one time will not necessarily work indefinitely. You'll have to play it by ear, and deal with each challenge with as much patience as possible.

QUESTION: When I find something she has hidden, I don't understand why she then accuses me of stealing it from her.

ANSWER: Remember, that's the disease talking. She has no real control over what her thoughts are. She will soon forget the incident, and you should, too. Don't argue with her, just move on to something else. Also, avoid leaving anything of importance around for her to take, so you don't have to search for it. Keep an area inaccessible to her, and put things away there directly, rather than putting them down to take care of later. Use a padlock or other device to block access to a closet, drawers, or even a whole room if you can.

QUESTION: What kind of research are they doing? How long will it be before they find a cure?

ANSWER: New research is started all the time. No one knows for sure how long it will be before a cure or prevention will be found. Every lead can result in a solution. One study compares twins who have Alzheimer's with their identical twins who do not. Unfortunately, research takes time. Still, there is progress. In 1993, tacrine (under the name of Cognex) was first put on the market, and the FDA approved donepezil hydrochloride (marketed under the name of Aricept) in 1996 to delay the progression of the disease. These drugs are effective when administered early on. They inhibit the enzyme that breaks down acetylcholine in the brain. Acetylcholine levels are low in Alzheimer patients, and since acetylcholine is an important neurotransmitter needed to form memory, delaying its breakdown is helpful to delay further cognitive loss (see chapter 1 for more details).

A relatively new product called galantamine has been used successfully in phase III drug trials. Over a one-year period, it maintained the cognitive scores of Alzheimer's patients with mild to moderate forms of the disease. That's great news, since the usual pattern is for memory and learning ability to decline as time goes by. So researchers are making progress, but slowly.

QUESTION: What kind of tests are there to identify different types of dementia?

ANSWER: Unlike many diseases that can be diagnosed by one or two tests, dementia usually requires several tests for a positive diagnosis. Alzheimer's disease is still often diagnosed through a process of elimination, ruling out one by one other conditions that might have some of the same symptoms as Alzheimer's (see chapter 1 for further details).

Any evaluation should start with a thorough physical exam, including laboratory tests. Since it's not uncommon for an elderly person to be disoriented because of nutritional deficiencies or the side effects of medication, questions to ferret out those potential causes must be included. A psychological exam should also be considered. An evaluation should include a CT scan and cognitive tests administered by a neurologist or someone else knowledgeable about mental function. A CT scan can eliminate other possible reasons for symptoms such as disorientation and confusion, memory loss, mood swings, and irrational behavior. The cognitive testing can be done quickly enough, asking questions that measure the patient's orientation to time and reality as well as verbal fluency. That would include, for example, asking what day it is, where the person is, and who the president of the United States is. Further questions would involve identifying simple objects and remembering a short list of items.

Different types of dementia have different characteristics, so it's important to see someone experienced in the field.

QUESTION: I've heard some vitamins can help treat dementia. Can they? What does alternative medicine have to offer?

ANSWER: Ginkgo biloba, vitamin E, lecithin, and estrogen have all been studied to see how they can help people with dementia. No study is conclusive, and different things help different people in different ways (see chapter 1). Consult with your physician. Although there is no cure, you can hope to delay and alleviate some of the symptoms.

As for alternative practitioners, they might suggest the food supplements listed above as well as a healthy lifestyle. They might recommend meditation and regular exercise as part of a healthy regimen. Such a lifestyle has been linked to better cognitive functioning. Researchers have concluded that, since exercise increases blood flow, it can preserve mental function by bringing more blood to the brain. (It was the lack of blood flow to certain areas of Newton's brain that caused his dementia.) Eating healthy food that is not overprocessed will contribute to a general sense of well-being. More and more studies emphasize the importance of eating lots of fruits and vegetables. All this may not make a big difference in your patient's functioning, but it won't hurt. Applying these guidelines to yourself will help you be stronger. So this is a good time to evaluate your own eating and exercise habits.

QUESTION: What kind of activities can my loved one participate in outside the home?
ANSWER: There are adult day care groups set up specifically for the benefit of dementia patients. Some meet once a week, some meet more often. There are full-day and half-day programs. Low-cost or no-cost counseling is also available. (See the resource guide that follows.)

QUESTION: What's available for me?
ANSWER: You are also eligible for counseling, with or without the patient. There are many support groups out there, too. Contact the Alzheimer's Association for further information. I urge you to seek out such a group. It will lighten your load and reduce your feeling of isolation.

QUESTION: A friend offered to help. What can I ask her to do? I don't want her to be turned off.

ANSWER: Ask her to sit with your loved one while you go out for a while or take a nap. Give her a supply of old photos and mementos, so she can reminisce with the patient, who can remember things from long ago much more easily than things from an hour ago. Also, let her play some music. Of course, if you are both comfortable with the idea, she could take your loved one to an appointment—and then you could take a bubble bath or something!

QUESTION: What are the statistics on Alzheimer's disease?
ANSWER: Alzheimer's disease affects 50 percent of those over eighty-five. A person with Alzheimer's lives an average of eight years after the diagnosis, but that means that some live a shorter amount of time, and some as long as twenty years. The average cost for caring for such a patient from the time of diagnosis to death is $174,000.

QUESTION: Is the government doing anything to help?
ANSWER: Congress is studying ways of helping pay for medication and care of dementia patients. The Alzheimer's Association has been asking to have Medicare policies changed so that people with dementia can be given more help, but no new guidelines have been established yet. Still, the federal government spent four hundred million dollars in 1999 for Alzheimer's research. This is a disease that affects so many people that our legislators want to see something done.

QUESTION: Where can I go for more information?
ANSWER: The Alzheimer's Association is dedicated to giving support to people suffering from dementing illnesses and their caregivers. They are also at the forefront of research to find a cure. Lists of their central locations and of other agencies in your area are in the resources section.

QUESTION: I worry that something might happen to me. I could get sick, or worse. What will become of my loved one if I'm not able to take care of him?

ANSWER: Just as parents make contingency plans for their small children when writing out their wills, you could prepare lists of names of people to contact in case of emergency. Speak to family members, even those far away. See who would be willing to take on the role of caregiver, even on a temporary basis. Also ask friends what their ideas are on the subject. If you think there is no one available to call on, talk to a social worker associated with your medical center, local hospital, or nearest mental health center. You can also ask your doctor for a referral.

Another list to prepare is one that contains suggested facilities that you have checked out so that your loved one would be taken care of properly if no individual could take over for you. This is all the more reason for you to check out local adult residences and nursing homes ahead of time (see chapter 5).

There are organizations that will give people guidance on long-term care. A sampling follows:

▷ National Family Caregivers Association
(800) 896-3650

Their twenty-dollar membership fee entitles caregivers to receive referrals and support.

▷ American Health Care Association
(202) 842-4444

They will send you a free brochure listing assisted living and nursing facilities that care for disabled adults throughout the fifty states.

▷ National Association for Homecare
(202) 547-7424

This is a trade association that represents over six thousand home-care agencies. They can help a caller choose a home-care provider.

Put in writing anything you think is important for someone else to know, be it about finances or details about handling your loved one. Keep the list in a handy place. Once you've done all this, you should have greater peace of mind and be able to devote yourself more completely to this most important role of yours, that of caregiver and handholder.

RESOURCES AND REFERENCES

When you're seeking help, you might not know where to turn. A visit to the public library or a search on the Web can give you answers, but you have precious little time to do research or to be put on hold when you call for general information. This section was created to make it easy for you to find assistance.

The Alzheimer's Association does a wonderful job of giving guidance and support to people dealing with dementia. But there are also many other organizations in this country that can be of help to you, the caregiver, and to your loved one. They offer a variety of services, depending on your location and needs.

Section A has several useful charts and forms that you can copy or use for reference. Section B lists resources for you to contact. If you have access to a computer, you can use the lists of useful Internet sites in section C. If you want to use your phone or you want to write instead of turning to a computer, there are lists of various providers and agencies. The agencies for the aging are listed state by state, in alphabetical order.

The different listings are accompanied by brief descriptions of what you can expect from them. I hope you find the help you need through these contacts.

A. CHARTS AND FORMS

Scheduling is crucial to survival at this time. You have to juggle so many regular events, from administering medication to going to see doctors, that it's easy to become bewildered. Add all the unexpected happenings, and you can be totally overwhelmed. That's why it would be a good idea for you to get a calendar with large boxes in which to write the appointments. A selection of calendars and date books is available in a variety of stores, including supermarkets.

On the following pages there are some helpful charts that you can't find easily in stores. You can enlarge them to suit your needs on most photocopying machines. Feel free to make as many copies as you think you'll need, and keep them on hand for regular use. It's worth the time it takes to fill out a chart, since the chart itself will be a time-saver. If you hang one or two schedules on the refrigerator, they can serve as guides and reminders for your patient, too.

DAILY SCHEDULE

TODAY IS: _____

7:00 A.M. _____

8:00 A.M. _____

9:00 A.M. _____

10:00 A.M. _____

11:00 A.M. _____

NOON _____

1:00 P.M. _____

2:00 P.M. _____

3:00 P.M. _____

4:00 P.M. _____

5:00 P.M. _____

6:00 P.M. _____

7:00 P.M. _____

8:00 P.M. _____

9:00 P.M. _____

10:00 P.M. _____

11:00 P.M. _____

REMINDERS: _____

_____

_____

_____

_____

DAILY MEDICATION CHART

NAME OF MEDICATION	NEEDED TODAY	TIME	TAKEN	NEEDED TODAY	TIME	TAKEN	NEEDED TODAY	TIME	TAKEN	NEEDED TODAY	TIME	TAKEN	NEEDED TODAY	TIME	TAKEN	NEEDED TODAY	TIME	TAKEN	NEEDED TODAY	TIME	TAKEN
1	Y/N	1 2 3 4		Y/N	1 2 3 4		Y/N	1 2 3 4		Y/N	1 2 3 4		Y/N	1 2 3 4		Y/N	1 2 3 4		Y/N	1 2 3 4	
2	Y/N	1 2 3 4		Y/N	1 2 3 4		Y/N	1 2 3 4		Y/N	1 2 3 4		Y/N	1 2 3 4		Y/N	1 2 3 4		Y/N	1 2 3 4	
3	Y/N	1 2 3 4		Y/N	1 2 3 4		Y/N	1 2 3 4		Y/N	1 2 3 4		Y/N	1 2 3 4		Y/N	1 2 3 4		Y/N	1 2 3 4	
4	Y/N	1 2 3 4		Y/N	1 2 3 4		Y/N	1 2 3 4		Y/N	1 2 3 4		Y/N	1 2 3 4		Y/N	1 2 3 4		Y/N	1 2 3 4	
5	Y/N	1 2 3 4		Y/N	1 2 3 4		Y/N	1 2 3 4		Y/N	1 2 3 4		Y/N	1 2 3 4		Y/N	1 2 3 4		Y/N	1 2 3 4	

In order for you to make decisions on financial matters, either to plan for Medicaid or to prepare your estate and your style of living, you need to have a picture of what you're worth. So, here are some charts that will help you to see where you stand. Once you've done the figuring, you will be more equipped to decide what, if anything, you should change. You'll be better able to plan for the future with the help of these charts.

PERSONAL FINANCIAL PICTURE:
DEBTS AS OF _____

	Name	Account #	Value
credit card balances:	_____	_____	_____
	_____	_____	_____
	_____	_____	_____
	_____	_____	_____
	_____	_____	_____
	_____	_____	_____
car loans:	_____	_____	_____
	_____	_____	_____
mortgages:	_____	_____	_____
other bank loans:	_____	_____	_____
	_____	_____	_____
	_____	_____	_____
private loans:	_____	_____	_____
	_____	_____	_____
other debts:	_____	_____	_____
	_____	_____	_____
	_____	_____	_____
	_____	_____	_____
	_____	_____	_____

Total debts: _____

PERSONAL FINANCIAL PICTURE:
ASSETS AS OF _____

	Name	Account #	Value
savings accounts:	_____	_____	_____
	_____	_____	_____
checking accounts:	_____	_____	_____
certificates of deposit:	_____	_____	_____
	_____	_____	_____
government bonds:	_____	_____	_____
	_____	_____	_____
municipal bonds:	_____	_____	_____
	_____	_____	_____
mutual funds:	_____	_____	_____
	_____	_____	_____
	_____	_____	_____
individual stocks:	_____	_____	_____
	_____	_____	_____
	_____	_____	_____
	_____	_____	_____
corporate bonds:	_____	_____	_____
	_____	_____	_____
real estate:	_____	_____	_____
cars:	_____	_____	_____
	_____	_____	_____
IRAs:	_____	_____	_____
401(k), etc.:	_____	_____	_____
life insurance:	_____	_____	_____
pension:	_____	_____	_____
Social Security:	_____	_____	_____
other:	_____	_____	_____
	_____	_____	_____
	_____	_____	_____
	_____	_____	_____

Total assets: _____

REGULAR LIVING EXPENSES

rent/mortgage: _____

utilities, repairs,
and maintenance: _____

car payments: _____

credit card debts: _____

medical and dental: _____

insurance premiums: _____

income taxes: _____

food: _____

transportation: _____

entertainment: _____

clothing—purchase: _____

clothing—upkeep: _____

legal: _____

travel: _____

gifts: _____

miscellaneous: _____

REGULAR INCOME

salary/pension: _____

Social Security: _____

interest/dividends: _____

other: _____

Total profit or loss: _____

The previous forms should help you put your finances in order. The following sample advance directives can give you an idea of how both you and your loved one can make your wishes known concerning end-of-life decisions.

These forms are valid for New York. Your state may have very different laws. You may want to consult an elder law attorney or call Partnership for Caring, Inc., at (800) 989-9455. Although you might not be able to use the same forms as New York's, Partnership for Caring can supply forms for every state. You could also use these advance directives as a springboard to a family discussion on the subject. It might make it easier to broach the topic.

The New York Health Care Proxy and Living Will is on the Internet at http://www.choices.org/pdfdocs/nydoc.pdf. There are other important resources on the Advance Directives page of this site: instructions, forms for every state, and important updates. The link to their Advanced Directives page is http://www.choices.org/ad.htm.

NEW YORK
HEALTH CARE PROXY

———————————————

(1) I, _____, hereby appoint:

(name)

PRINT NAME,
HOME ADDRESS
AND
TELEPHONE
NUMBER OF
YOUR AGENT

_____

(name, home address and telephone number of agent)

_____

as my health care agent to make any and all health care decisions for me, except to the extent that I state otherwise.

This Health Care Proxy shall take effect in the event I become unable to make my own health care decisions.

(2) Optional instructions: I direct my agent to make health care decisions in accord with my wishes and limitations as stated below, or as he or she otherwise knows.

(Unless your agent knows your wishes about artificial nutrition and hydration [feeding tubes], your agent will not be allowed to make decisions about artificial nutrition and hydration.)

PRINT NAME, HOME ADDRESS AND TELEPHONE NUMBER OF YOUR ALTERNATE AGENT

(3) Name of substitute or fill-in agent if the person I appoint above is unable, unwilling or unavailable to act as my health care agent.

_____

(name, home address and telephone number of alternate agent)

_____

ENTER A DURATION OR A CONDITION (IF ANY)

(4) Unless I revoke it, this proxy shall remain in effect indefinitely, or until the date or condition I have stated below. This proxy shall expire (specific date or conditions, if desired): _____

_____

SIGN AND DATE THE DOCUMENT AND PRINT YOUR ADDRESS

(5) Signature __ _____ Date _____

Address _____

WITNESSING PROCEDURE

Statement by Witnesses (must be 18 or older)

I declare that the person who signed this document appeared to execute the proxy willingly and free from duress. He or she signed (or asked another to sign for him or her) this document in my presence. I am not the person appointed as proxy by this document.

YOUR WITNESSES MUST SIGN AND PRINT THEIR ADDRESSES

Witness 1 _____ _____

Address _____

Witness 2 _____

Address _____

NEW YORK LIVING WILL

This Living Will has been prepared to conform to the law in the State of New York, as set forth in the case In re Westchester County Medical Center, 72 N.Y.2d 517 (1988). In that case the Court established the need for "clear and convincing" evidence of a patient's wishes and stated that the "ideal situation is one in which the patient's wishes were expressed in some form of writing, perhaps a 'living will.'"

PRINT YOUR NAME

I, _____, being of sound mind, make this statement as a directive to be followed if I become permanently unable to participate in decisions regarding my medical care. These instructions reflect my firm and settled commitment to decline medical treatment under the circumstances indicated below:

I direct my attending physician to withhold or withdraw treatment that merely prolongs my dying, if I should be in an **incurable or irreversible mental or physical condition with no reasonable expectation of recovery,** including but not limited to: (a) **a terminal condition;** (b) **a permanently unconscious condition;** or (c) **a minimally conscious condition in which I am permanently unable to make decisions or express my wishes.**

I direct that my treatment be limited to measures to keep me comfortable and to relieve pain, including any pain that might occur by withholding or withdrawing treatment.

While I understand that I am not legally required to be specific about future treatments **if I am in the condition(s) described above I feel especially strongly about the following forms of treatment:**

CROSS OUT ANY STATEMENTS THAT DO NOT REFLECT YOUR WISHES

    I do not want cardiac resuscitation.
    I do not want mechanical respiration.
    I do not want artificial nutrition and hydration.
    I do not want antibiotics.

    However, I **do want** maximum pain relief, even if it may hasten my death.

ADD PERSONAL INSTRUCTIONS (IF ANY)

Other directions:

These directions express my legal right to refuse treatment, under the law of New York. I intend my instructions to be carried out, unless I have rescinded them in a new writing or by clearly indicating that I have changed my mind.

SIGN AND DATE THE DOCUMENT AND PRINT YOUR ADDRESS

Signed _____ Date _____

Address _____

WITNESSING PROCEDURE

I declare that the person who signed this document appeared to execute the living will willingly and free from duress. He or she signed (or asked another to sign for him or her) this document in my presence.

YOUR WITNESSES MUST SIGN AND PRINT THEIR ADDRESSES

Witness 1 _____

Address _____

Witness 2 _____

Address _____

© 1996
CHOICE IN DYING, INC.

Courtesy of **Choice In Dying, Inc.**
1035 30th Street, NW Washington, DC 20007 800-989-9455

6/96

The first section of this appendix lists agencies that will give you advice and information about the disease, and help you obtain a variety of supplies. The second section is organized by state, and lists agencies for the aging in each state. In both sections, you'll find specific information about what each organization offers. Some spokespeople were more detailed in their answers to my questions than others. That is not a reflection on the quality of service they offer. The last section of this appendix gives information about Internet sites so that you or someone you know can find what you need without having to wade through the countless listings connected to Alzheimer's. There are specifics about each Web site to simplify your quest.

Nationwide Agencies for the Elderly

The first call you might want to make is to the central office of the Alzheimer's Association. They will refer you to your local chapter. You can contact them for guidance even if your loved one has a form of dementia other than Alzheimer's.

▷ Alzheimer's Association
919 N. Michigan Ave., Suite 1100
Chicago, IL 60611
(800) 621-0379 or in Illinois (800) 572-6037

The National Institute on Aging's information office can help you better understand the disease.

▷ National Institute on Aging
31 Center Dr., Room 5C27
Bethesda, MD 20892
(301) 496-1752

Care Catalog Services has a full range of home health care equipment for the elderly.

▷ Care Catalog Services
1877 NE Seventh Ave.
Portland, OR 97212
(503) 288-8174 or (800) 443-7091 to place orders

The American Health Assistance Foundation (AHAF) is devoted to funding scientific research on Alzheimer's disease as well as other age-related degenerative diseases. AHAF also has an Alzheimer's Family Relief Program that provides financial assistance to Alzheimer's patients who are in need. They provide $500 cash grants to qualified Alzheimer's patients. In addition, AHAF will send you free information on Alzheimer's upon request.

▷ American Health Assistance Foundation
15825 Shady Grove Rd., Suite 140
Rockville, MD 20850
(301) 948-3244 or (800) 437-2423

The American Association of Retired Persons (AARP) is a nonprofit organization that sponsors a wide range of educational programs, a computerized bibliographic database, publications, and a mail-order pharmacy.

▷ American Association of Retired Persons
601 E St. NW
Washington, DC 20049
(202) 434-AARP (2277)

The American Dietetic Association is a professional society of dietitians. They work in health care settings, in schools, and in day care centers, as well as in business. They provide nutrition services and dietary counseling. You can call for their publications or to find a registered dietitian in your community.

▷ American Dietetic Association
216 W. Jackson Blvd., Suite 800
Chicago, IL 60606
(312) 899-0040

The American Health Association is a professional organization that represents the interests of licensed nursing homes and long-term-care facilities to Congress and other groups. Contact them to have information on long-term care sent to you.

▷ American Health Association
1201 L St. NW
Washington, DC 20005
(202) 842-4444

The American Psychological Association offers counseling for mental, emotional, or behavioral problems. State chapters will also help you find a psychologist for consultation.

▷ American Psychological Association
750 First St. NE
Washington, DC 20002
(202) 336-5500

B'nai Brith International is a voluntary service organization. Members of local chapters visit and care for the sick and offer programs to help the poor, widowed, and elderly. They are at:

▷ B'nai Brith International
1640 Rhode Island Ave. NW
Washington, DC 20036
(202) 857-6600

Catholic Charities USA offers many services for the elderly. They provide counseling, homemaker and health care services, institutional care, public-access programs, health clinics, and emergency assistance and shelter.

▷ Catholic Charities USA
1731 King St., Suite 200
Alexandria, VA 22314
(703) 549-1390

The Center for the Study of Aging will send you materials on aging, health, fitness, and wellness. They also offer Alzheimer's patients referrals to other agencies.

▷ Center for the Study of Aging
706 Madison Ave.
Albany, NY 12208-3695
(518) 465-6927

Children of Aging Parents (CAPS) gives information and emotional support to caregivers. This organization also offers referrals to attorneys, support groups, caregiving facilities, nursing homes, and counseling. You can send for their booklet that covers all aspects of caregiving.

▷ Children of Aging Parents
1609 Woodbourne Rd., Suite 302-A
Levittown, PA 19057
(215) 945-6900

Help for Incontinent People, Inc., is a patient-advocacy group. It is a good source of information and support to the public and health professionals about the causes, prevention, diagnosis, treatments, and management of incontinence. You can call their toll-free number or send for their publications for more information.

▷ Help for Incontinent People, Inc.
P.O. Box 544
Union, SC 29379
(803) 579-7900 or (800) BLADDER (252-3337)

The Medicare Choices Hotline provides up-to-date information about Medicare, health plan options in your community, available managed

care plans and supplemental insurance. Callers can talk to a representative in English or Spanish from 9 A.M. to 4:30 P.M. Monday
through Friday.

▷ Medicare Choices Hotline
(800) 633-4227

The National Association of Area Agencies on Aging (NAAAA) is a
private nonprofit organization. It offers services such as transportation, legal aid, nutrition programs, housekeeping, senior center activities, employment counseling, and referral programs.

▷ National Association of Area Agencies on Aging
927 15th St. NW
Washington, DC 20005
(202) 296-8130

The National Association for Home Care will help you find a home
care agency and will provide assistance in searching for solutions to
your home care problems.

▷ National Association for Home Care
519 C St. NE
Washington, DC 20002
(202) 547-7424

The National Council on the Aging, Inc., is a nonprofit organization
that provides information, consultation services, and research on aging.

▷ National Council on the Aging, Inc.
409 Third St. SW, Suite 200
Washington, DC 20024
(202) 479-1200

The National Family Caregivers Association is a nonprofit organization that serves family caregivers with helpful tips and support. They
don't focus on any one disease, but they do have referrals and helpful booklets to assist in finding an appropriate organization to meet
your individual needs.

▷ National Family Caregivers Association
9223 Longbranch Parkway
Silver Spring, MD 20901-3642
(301) 942-6430 or (301) 949-3638

The National Hospice Organization provides referrals and information on hospice services and care.

▷ National Hospice Organization
1901 N. Moore St., Suite 901
Arlington, VA 22209
(800) 658-8898 or (703) 243-5900

The National Institute of Neurologic Disorders and Stroke has free publications on neurologic diseases, including Alzheimer's and other dementias. They also offer helpful phone numbers for Alzheimer's patients and will send you an information booklet.

▷ National Institute of Neurologic Disorders and Stroke
Information Office
Building 31, Room 8A06
9000 Rockville Pike
Bethesda, MD 20892
(301) 496-5751

The National Institute on Aging Information Center is a federal agency that provides free materials to the public, including fact sheets, pamphlets, and reports on Alzheimer's disease, aging, medical care, nutrition, safety, and exercise.

▷ National Institute on Aging Information Center
P.O. Box 8057
Gaithersburg, MD 20898-8057
(800) 222-2225

The United Way of America is an association with local agencies in cities across the United States. They offer support, social services, and public assistance programs for the elderly. You can contact the main agency to find out about what's available locally.

▷ United Way of America
701 N. Fairfax St.
Alexandria, VA 22314-2045
(703) 836-7100

The Visiting Nurse Association of America offers information and referral services for physical, occupational, and speech therapy as well as general nursing. It also has an adult day care center, wellness clinic, and meals-on-wheels program.

▷ Visiting Nurse Association of America
3801 E. Florida Ave., Suite 206
Denver, CO 80210
(800) 426-2547

State-by-State Agencies for the Elderly

There is an Elder Care Locator at (800) 677-1116. They can give you information about services available to the elderly anywhere in the country, but you may have to be on hold for quite a while.

In addition, you may want to refer to the following resource list of support agencies throughout the United States. Some can offer more than others, and some are more helpful than others. It's certainly worth a phone call to find out what's available near you. Many of these agencies move unexpectedly, and their area codes can be changed even if they don't move. You may have to be persistent, be on hold, or call back when the line isn't busy. I found that the best time to get through was in the late morning.

Most of the funding comes from our tax dollars, so don't hesitate to avail yourself of the services offered.

▷ Alabama
Jefferson City Commission on Aging
3712 Fourth Ave. S.
Birmingham, AL 35222
(205) 592-0413
They offer Meals-on-Wheels among other services.

▷ Alaska
Alaska Commission on Aging
P.O. Box 110209
Juneau, AK 99811
(907) 465-3250

Division of Senior Services
3601 C St., Suite 310
Anchorage, AK 99503
(907) 269-3654
They will refer you to the correct branch of the Division of Senior Services, which can offer long-term-care coordination, among other services.

▷ Arizona
Aging and Adult Administration
Department of Economic Security
1366 E. Thomas Rd., Suite 108
Phoenix, AZ 85014
(602) 542-4446
Ask for their "Senior Help Line." It can arrange for home delivered meals, bathing, respite care, and more.

▷ Arkansas
Division of Aging and Adult Services,
Arkansas Department of Human Services
P.O. Box 14137, Slot 1412
Seventh and Main Sts.

Little Rock, AR 72203
(501) 682-2441

They will refer you to your area's agency on aging for specific information on what's available near you.

▷ California
Department of Aging
1600 K St.
Sacramento, CA 95814
(916) 322-5290 or in California (800) 510-2020

They will refer you to one of the thirty-three area agencies on aging in fifty-eight cities that offer services such as meals and counseling on health insurance.

▷ Colorado
Aging and Adult Service, Department of Social Services
1575 Sherman St., Ground Floor
Denver, CO 80203
(303) 866-2800

They offer a great variety of support, including Meals-on-Wheels, in-home and respite care, and counseling.

▷ Connecticut
Department on Aging
10 Middle St.
Bridgeport, CT 06604
(203) 333-9288

They can put you in touch with their statewide respite program, and they will also give you information about other available services.

▷ Delaware
Division of Aging and Adults with Physical Disabilities
1901 N. DuPont Highway
New Castle, DE 19720
(302) 421-6791 or in Delaware (800) 464-4357

You can call the Delaware government helpline at (800) 273-9500 to get in touch with their referral service and receive information from their database.

▷ District of Columbia
Office on Aging
441 Fourth St. NW, Suite 900
Washington, DC 20001
(202) 724-5626 or (202) 727-8367

Their long-term-care specialist is trained in case management, and will help you find the appropriate day care and home care services, and will arrange for caregiver advice, counseling, and legal services.

▷ Florida
Department of Elder Affairs
4040 Esplanade Way, Suite 152
Tallahassee, FL 32399
(850) 414-2000
They offer a spectrum of care in which they interact with a large network of agencies throughout the state. The Elder Helpline can arrange for many services, which vary from region to region. Here's a sampling: Meals-on-Wheels, nutritional and other counseling, transportation, financial advice, in-home and respite care, and adult day care.

▷ Georgia
Division of Aging Services
Department of Human Resources
2 Peachtree St. NE, 36th Floor
Atlanta, GA 30303
(404) 657-5258
Depending on the county you live in, you will be referred to one of their twelve area agencies, some of which offer respite care. They will evaluate your eligibility for these services.

▷ Hawaii
Executive Office on Aging
250 S. Hotel St., Suite 109
Honolulu, HI 96813
(808) 586-0100
They have an Alzheimer's representative who can give you advice and guidance.

▷ Idaho
Commission on Aging
3380 Americana Terr., Suite 120
Boise, ID 83706
(208) 334-3833
They administer the funding for six area agencies and will refer you to the correct one.

▷ Illinois
Department on Aging
421 E. Capital Ave., #100
Springfield, IL 62701
(217) 785-2870
Their senior helpline staff will send you a booklet, "Choices for Care," from which you can select which community care, adult care, and homemaker services you want.

▷ Indiana

Division of Aging Services, Department of Human Services
P.O. Box 7083
402 W. Washington St., Room w454
Indianapolis, IN 46207
(317) 232-7020

They offer in-home services, nutrition advice, and advocacy.

▷ Iowa

Department of Elder Affairs
200 Tenth St., Clemens Building, Third Floor
Des Moines, IA 50309
(515) 281-5187 or (800) 532-3213

If the patient is living at home, they will refer you to agencies that can
help you with your specific request. If the patient is in a facility and
there are problems, their ombudsman will help you resolve them.

▷ Kansas

Department on Aging
New England Building
503 S. Kansas Ave.
Topeka, KS 66603
(785) 296-4986

They can direct you to the Alzheimer's helpline at (800) 432-3535. They
know coordinators of Alzheimer's associations throughout the state.

▷ Kentucky

Office of Aging Services
Cabinet for Families and Children
Commonwealth of Kentucky
275 E. Main St., 5WA
Frankfort, KY 40621
(502) 564-6930

They will put you in contact with an agency in your neighborhood that
can arrange for such things as support groups, respite, and day care.

▷ Louisiana

Governor's Office of Elderly Affairs
P.O. Box 80374
Baton Rouge, LA 70898
(225) 342-7100

They will refer you to your local "parish" that can arrange for a variety of services such as home meals and congregate meals, transportation to medical services, recreational activities, homemaker
services, and personal care.

▷ Maine
Bureau of Elder and Adult Services
Department of Human Services
35 Anthony Ave.
State House, Station #11
Augusta, ME 04333
(207) 624-5335

Services are offered through five area agencies. They can put you in contact with the right agency for a variety of services like respite care.

▷ Maryland
Maryland Department of Aging
State Office Building, Room 1007
301 W. Preston St.
Baltimore, MD 21201
(410) 767-1100

They will refer you to the correct information and assistance program in your area.

▷ Massachusetts
Massachusetts Executive Office of Elder Affairs
1 Ashburton Place, 5th Floor
Boston, MA 02108
(617) 727-7750

They will refer you to the right Alzheimer's Association helpline.

▷ Michigan
Michigan Office of Services to the Aging
611 W. Ottawa
N. Ottawa Tower, 3rd Floor
P.O. Box 30676
Lansing, MI 48909
(517) 373-8230

They will refer you to your local Alzheimer's Association and to one of the sixteen regional area agencies on aging.

▷ Minnesota
Minnesota Board on Aging
444 Lafayette Rd.
St. Paul, MN 55155
(651) 296-2738, (651) 297-5459, or (800) 333-2433

Ask for their Senior Linkage to find out about a great variety of services, from meals to support groups. They also offer caregiver support through their Alzheimer's Section, (800) 232-0851.

▷ Mississippi
Division of Aging and Adult Services
750 N. State St.
Jackson, MS 39202
(601) 359-4925

They offer community-based case management. They will give you the help you need to maintain your loved one at home, and then, when it becomes necessary, they can refer you to nursing homes in your area that specialize in Alzheimer's care.

▷ Missouri
Division on Aging
Department of Social Services
P.O. Box 1337
615 Howerton Ct.
Jefferson City, MO 65102
(573) 751-3082

They give advice on nutrition and help with transportation. They have legal services, in-home help, and long-term-care facilities. They also work closely with the five Alzheimer's Association chapters in the state, which offer support groups and training.

▷ Montana
Senior and Long-Term Care Division
Department of Public Health and Human Services
P.O. Box 4210
111 Sanders, Room 211
Helena, MT 59620
(406) 444-7788 or (406) 444-7782

They administer Older American Act funds and contract with 11 area agencies on aging and 175 senior centers. These centers offer Meals-on-Wheels and can arrange for respite care. Local Alzheimer's Association chapters refer people to support groups, doctors, and home health care agencies.

▷ Nebraska
Department of Health and Human Services
Division on Aging
P.O. Box 95044
1343 M St.
Lincoln, NE 68509
(402) 471-2307

They will refer you to one of the eight area agencies. Each one offers different services, including a care management program. This program involves having someone come to your home and assess your situation. Then they can give you guidance on how to get different kinds of help, including financial aid.

▷ Nevada
Nevada Division for Aging Services
Department of Human Resources
State Mail Room Complex
3416 Goni Rd., Bldg. D #132
Carson City, NV 89706
(775) 687-4210

They can arrange for you to get Meals-on-Wheels from a local senior center, and they also offer home help and personal care.

▷ New Hampshire
Division of Elderly and Adult Services
District State Office Park South
129 Pleasant St., Brown Bldg. #1
Concord, NH 03301
(603) 271-4680

Through one of their twelve offices, they will offer home community care or long-term care, and they will help you deal with nursing homes.

▷ New Jersey
New Jersey Division of Senior Affairs
Department of Health and Senior Services
P.O. Box 807
Trenton, NJ 08625
(609) 588-3141, (609) 588-3274, or (800) 792-8820

They can arrange for rebates for things like hearing aids. They also give advice on SSI (Supplemental Security Income).

▷ New Mexico
State Agency on Aging
La Villa Rivera Bldg.
228 E. Palace Ave., Ground Floor
Santa Fe, NM 87501
(505) 827-7640

Ask to talk to an Alzheimer's counselor, who will tell you about a variety of benefits. The Assistance Corps, which helps all seniors, has special resources for dementia patients.

▷ New York
New York State Office for the Aging
2 Empire State Plaza
Albany, NY 12223
(518) 474-5731 or (800) 342-9871

They have a referral information service for people in different counties throughout the state. Ask for their resource guide, which lists such services as home health care and Heat Energy Assistance Program (HEAP).

▷ North Carolina

Department of Health and Human Services
Division of Aging
Caller Box 29531
Raleigh, NC 27626
(919) 733-3983

They will refer you to Services Operations that can arrange for home care, day care, or nutrition services. They also have information on elder rights.

▷ North Dakota

Aging Services Division
Department of Human Services
600 S. Second St., Suite 1C
Bismarck, ND 58504
(701) 328-8910 or (800) 451-8693

They oversee home-based and community-based services like meals and transportation. They also have an ombudsman program for nursing home and assisted living facilities.

▷ Ohio

Ohio Department of Aging
50 W. Broad St., 9th Floor
Columbus, OH 43215
(614) 466-5500

They will refer you to your area agency on aging, which might arrange for you to have Meals-on-Wheels and help in the home with cleaning or health care.

▷ Oklahoma

Aging Services Division
Department of Human Services
312 NE 28th St.
Oklahoma City, OK 73105
(405) 521-2281

They will refer you to one of their eleven area agencies, which offer a variety of services such as home health care, household help, and food.

▷ Oregon

Senior and Disabled Services Division
500 Summer St. NE, Second Floor
Salem, OR 97310
(503) 945-5811

Depending on where you live, a variety of services are available. Call for details.

▷ Pennsylvania
Pennsylvania Department of Aging
Commonwealth of Pennsylvania
555 Walnut St., 5th Floor
Harrisburg, PA 17101
(717) 783-1550

If you are over the age of sixty, you will be put in contact with one of fifty-two area agencies on aging that might offer food, transportation, and home health care.

▷ Rhode Island
Department of Elderly Affairs
160 Pine St.
Providence, RI 02903
(401) 222-2858

They offer home and community care, which includes an eating program and pharmaceutical programs. Ask for their booklet to get more details.

▷ South Carolina
Office of Senior and Long-Term Care Services
Department of Health and Human Services
P.O. Box 8206
Columbia, SC 29202
(803) 898-2501

This Medicare branch of the state government will refer you to your county office for help. Core services include transportation, home companion and respite care, meals, and case management.

▷ South Dakota
Office of Adult Services and Aging
Richard F. Kneip Bldg.
700 Governors Dr.
Pierre, SD 57501
(605) 773-3656

You can arrange for home care, personal care, respite care, and assisted living through them.

▷ Tennessee
Commission on Aging
Andrew Jackson Building, 9th Floor
500 Deaderick St.
Nashville, TN 37243
(615) 741-2056

They provide funding for district agencies on aging and will refer you to their informational and referral program for such things as legal assistance, transportation, and meals.

▷ Texas

Texas Department on Aging
4900 N. Lamar, 4th Floor
Austin, TX 78751
(512) 424-6840

They fund the different area agencies on aging. These agencies dispense various services, depending on your locale.

▷ Utah

Division of Aging and Adult Services
Box 45500
120 N. 200 West
Salt Lake City, UT 84145
(801) 538-3910

They will refer you to different agencies to arrange for Meals-on-Wheels, transportation, and adult day care centers.

▷ Vermont

Vermont Department of Aging and Disabilities
Waterbury Complex
103 S. Main St.
Waterbury, VT 05671
(802) 241-2400

Ask to speak to a program staff member who can arrange for an attendant or an independent living facility. They can also guide you on their Metropolitan Waiver Program.

▷ Virginia

Virginia Department for the Aging
1600 Forest Ave., Suite 102
Richmond, VA 23229
(804) 662-9333

They will refer you to one of the twenty-five area agencies on aging that offer services ranging from transportation to adult day care to home-delivered meals and in-home care.

▷ Washington

Aging and Adult Services Administration
Department of Social and Health Services
P.O. Box 45600
Olympia, WA 98504
(360) 493-2500

The Home and Community Services division will help you with a variety of services. They will also give you information on nursing homes and boarding homes.

▷ West Virginia
West Virginia Bureau of Senior Services
Holly Grove Bldg. 10
1900 Kanawha Blvd. E
Charleston, WV 25305
(304) 558-3317

Services are provided by the local county office closest to you. They can include transportation, food, and home health care.

▷ Wisconsin
Bureau of Aging and Long-Term Care Resources
Department of Health and Family Services
P.O. Box 7851
Madison, WI 53707
(608) 266-2536

They will send you a brochure that explains the services available. They include counseling, food, transportation, and home health care.

▷ Wyoming
Office on Aging, Department of Health
6101 Yellowstone Rd., Room 259B
Cheyenne, WY 82002
(307) 777-7986

They will refer you to the appropriate Division of Family Services office. Each office gives advice on Medicaid, food, and transportation. Some offer counseling as well.

C. INTERNET RESOURCES

The Internet is a valuable source of information. However, there is no regulatory agency to assure that all the statements are truthful. Also, there is no guarantee that a given Web site will be in existence a month later. Keeping that in mind, if you have access to the Internet, you can gather a lot of helpful information. If you do a keyword search on "Alzheimer's," you'll find at least five hundred Web sites. To spare you from sorting through all these data, I've put together the following list of some of the sites you might want to take a look at.

Alzheimer's Association

Although the Alzheimer's Association has several Web sites, there isn't one posted for every state. If you cannot find your state's Web site, contact the main Alzheimer's Association Web site: http://www.alz.org. This site contains five links: facts on Alzheimer's, taking care of your patient and yourself, medical issues, research, and information about the association itself.

—— Alzheimer's Association local chapters: http://www.alz.org/chapters

   Visit this page to find out about an Alzheimer's Association chapter near you.

—— Alzheimer's Association, Cleveland Area Chapter: http://www.alzclv.org

   It is easy to get data on this Web site, which is equipped with information about the top ten warning signs of Alzheimer's, a telephone helpline, details about the Safe Return Program, the Respite Reimbursement Program, and Home Helper's Registry. It also has an e-mail address for questions and comments, along with a phone number and mailing address.

—— Alzheimer's Association, Greater Chicagoland Chapter: http://www.alzchi.org

   This Web site has referrals that give support to Alzheimer's patients, family members, and caregivers.

—— Alzheimer's Association, Greater Cincinnati Chapter: http://www.alz.org/chapters/template/grtrcinc

   This Web site is organized by volunteers. They explore possible preventions, cures, and treatments for Alzheimer's disease.

—— Alzheimer's Association, Northern Virginia Chapter: http://www.alz-nova.org

   This Web site provides information on programs and services for families and caregivers. It also educates the general public and health professionals about Alzheimer's disease.

—— Alzheimer's Association, San Francisco, Greater Bay Area Chapter: http://www.alzsf.org

   The San Francisco Alzheimer's Association site has information about support services, advocacy, and research on Alzheimer's disease and related disorders.

—— Alzheimer's Association, Tampa Bay Chapter:
http://www.alz-tbc.org
    This Web site has information about services and local programs
for patients and families with Alzheimer's disease.

—— Alzheimer's Association, Victoria:
http://www.vicnet.net.au/vicnet/community/alzheim/index.html
    This association's primary goal is to enhance the quality of life
for caregivers and their dementia patients. Through this Web site you
can find information about dementia and ways to get free counseling services. They also offer free "educational training" for caretakers.
In addition, it has a library as well as phone numbers and addresses
for more information. The best thing about this Web site is that it's
from Australia, offering information one would not normally have
access to in the U.S.

—— Alzheimer's Disease Society, Durham and Chester, UK:
http://www.users.zetnet.co.uk/durham.ads
    The United Kingdom (England) branch provides information, care-
giver support, and access to respite day care and drop-in facilities.

—— Alzheimer's Society—Société Alzheimer:
http://www.alzheimer.ca
    This is a national nonprofit organization developed to help Cana-
dians affected by Alzheimer's disease. It lists the latest information
on Alzheimer's care and research. It also offers support and forums
for caregivers and physicians.

Facts and Background Information

—— Ability Organization:
http://www.ability.org.uk/alzheime.html
    Their slogan is "See the ability, not the disability." This Web site
has a link page of at least sixty resources in alphabetical order. They
link to almost anything that can connect or help with Alzheimer's,
from caregiving to nursing homes to books and associations.

—— About Alzheimer's:
http://nymemory.org
    This site lists treatments of Alzheimer's disease. It also has fre-
quently asked questions and their answers.

—— Allexperts Alzheimer's Question and Answer:
http://www.allexperts.com
    This is a Web site worth visiting. Doctors and other specialists
answer your questions about Alzheimer's disease one-on-one. There
is no fee.

—— Alois Alzheimer's Center:
http://www.alois.com

This site tells about the Alois Alzheimer's Center and gives contact information on care, treatment, and a study of Alzheimer's disease.

—— Alzheimer's.com:
http://www.alzheimers.com

This site presents a comprehensive online resource that is updated daily. It has the latest news and information about Alzheimer's.

—— Alzheimer's Disease:
http://encarta.msn.com/find/search.asp?search=alzheimers

This is a complete Web site with almost anything you need to know about Alzheimer's, its symptoms, abnormalities, causes, diagnosis, treatment, and caretaking. It recommends books for more information and gives you the latest updated articles from health science magazines.

—— Alzheimer's Disease at Suite 101.com:
http://www.suite101.com/welcome.cfm/alzheimers_disease

This page consists of biweekly articles about Alzheimer's disease, updated links, informal polls, and discussions with doctors. The articles are a good resource because they are frequently updated. You can check this Web site for new information.

—— Alzheimer's Disease Education and Referral Center (ADEAR):
http://www.alzheimers.org

ADEAR is a service of the National Institute on Aging and National Institutes of Health. It offers information on Alzheimer's disease research, clinical trials, and publications. It has a bibliographic database and links to other federal resources.

—— Alzheimer's Disease Mini Information Sheet:
http://ninds.nih.gov/patients/disorder/alzheim/alz

The National Institutes of Health puts out facts about the illness on this Web site.

—— Alzheimer's Disease Resource Center:
http://www.healingwell.com/alzheimers

This site contains medical news, information, articles, book titles, message boards, news groups, and links to related sites.

—— Alzheimer's Disease/Senility:
http://www.crha-health.ab.ca/hlthconn/items/alz.htm

This Web site outlines deterioration of brain function in those past sixty. It also gives suggestions to caregivers.

—— Alzheimer's Resource Center:
http://www.mayohealth.org/mayo/common/htm/alzheimers.htm

Mayo Clinic Health Oasis experts offer information, explanations, and advice about treatment and care for people with Alzheimer's disease.

— Dementia:
http://www.alzforum.org/members

This Web site outlines different types of dementia. It helps clarify the confusion between Alzheimer's and other dementias.

— Dementia Symptoms:
http://www.merck.com/pubs/mm_geriatrics

This site gives an overview and fact sheet on dementia.

— Dr. Koop:
http://www.drkoop.com

This is a Web site created by Dr. C. Everett Koop, who is known for his motto, "The best prescription is knowledge." His Web site has a whole page dedicated to Alzheimer's. It offers a library/encyclopedia link, health news, family health, health and wellness, and community links. The Web site is especially good if you want to find out about recent drug treatments and studies.

— Dr. Michael Rebhan:
http://www.uni-hohenheim.de/~rebhan/index.html

In this site, a biologist/neurologist lays out his latest research, term papers, and treatments on Alzheimer's.

— Elder Network:
http://www.senior.com

This is a general Web site for seniors. It guides you on eating, reading, and meeting. It also has medical information.

— Facts on Alzheimer's:
http://www.alzheimers.org/pub/adfact.html

This site presents a number of facts about the illness.

— Facts on Alzheimer's Disease:
http://www.alzheimers.org/pubs/adfact.html

This site offers information and facts on the illness.

— Genetics of Alzheimer's Disease:
http://www.alzheiemrs.org/genefact.html

In this site you'll find studies on the genetics of familial Alzheimer's disease.

— Neurological Disorders:
http://healthlink.mcw.edu/neurological-disorders

This Web site is created by physicians from the Medical College of Wisconsin. It gives information on neurological disorders.

— Resources on Alzheimer's Disease:
http://www.alzheimersbooks.com/Resources.html

This site describes Alzheimer's videotape resources.

— SeniorLink Home Page:
http://www.seniorlink.com

This site offers general elder care resources for seniors. It gives access to elder care professionals, programs, providers, facilities, and agencies.

— University of Washington Alzheimer's Disease Research Center:
http://depts.washington.edu/adrcweb

At this site, they have information for researchers, health care providers, and families.

— U.S. Resources: Alzheimer's Disease, etc.:
http://www.aoa.dhhs.gov/jpost/us-ad.html

Put together by the Administration on Aging, this site offers resources related to Alzheimer's disease and other dementias. It has links to discussion groups and listservs. It also contains information about research in the United States and other countries.

— Wisconsin Alzheimer's Institute:
http://www.medsch.wisc.edu/wai

The Wisconsin Alzheimer's Institute helps with research, education, training, program development, and advocacy information.

Sources of Help and Inspiration for Caregivers

— Alzheimer's.com Community Board and Support:
http://alzheimers.com/cgi-bin/affinity

This site has notes from hundreds of caregivers on techniques they have found useful for caring for loved ones with Alzheimer's.

— Alzheimer's Disease Caregivers Speak Out:
http://www.chpublishers.com

This Web site is a caregiver-to-caregiver guide for understanding Alzheimer's and dealing with your patient.

— Alzheimer's Disease Support Group:
http://www.supportgroup.com

This Web site is organized so you can find support groups and organizations in your state. There are links to government information sites, to various resources, and to information about alternative therapies. Caregivers speak out on the personal pages. You can be put on a mailing list for more specific information, like frequently asked questions and their answers.

—— Caregiver-information.com:
http://caregiver-information.com
This site gives information for those caring for people with Alzheimer's disease, stroke, or traumatic brain injury.

—— Caregiver Support:
http://www.nymemory.org
People who have been caretakers give information on techniques for caregiving, frequently asked questions, and an overview of their experiences.

—— Resources on Alzheimer's Disease:
http://www.alzheimerbooks.com
This Web site is actually a link to a list of resources like the following: ALZwell Alzheimer's Caregiver's Page is a Web site dedicated to helping the caregiver. It is equipped with information escapes and outlets. It even has a "story of the day" to cheer up caregivers and give them a well-needed smile. Other features are a link to caregiving chat rooms, a resource library, "What's New Every Day" link, and even a space for new people to share their experience and vent—it's called the "Anger Wall," a way for caregivers to let out the anger that has built up that day. The Cognitive Neurology and Alzheimer's Disease Center (CN-ADC) offers a Web site with information on the latest research and discoveries in the field. This includes information on the "why" and "how" of Alzheimer's and ways to help patients with brain diseases. Friendly4Seniors is a Web page that helps seniors with information, resources, services, and support groups.

—— Time Slips:
http://www.timeslips.org/go.html
This site offers stories told by patients with Alzheimer's disease.

—— What is Sundowning?
http://highlander.cbnet.ns.ca/asoc/care/sundown.html
This site is maintained by the Alzheimer's Society of Ottawa-Carelton. They describe sundowning and suggest ways to alleviate the problem.

—— A Year to Remember:
http://www.zarcrom.com
This site provides Alzheimer's disease information and shares a personal story through poetry, photos, and a caregiver's journal. It also has a message board.

Research, Medical, and Nutritional Information

—— About Estrogen, Memory and Menopause:
http://www.nymemory.org/devig/menmemandmoo.html

This site has frequently asked questions about memory and cognitive loss due to estrogen deficits.

—— Alternative Natural Treatment of Alzheimer's Disease:
http://www.meditopia.com/alzhome.html

This site relays alternative natural treatments of Alzheimer's disease using Asian medicine.

—— Alzheimer's Disease:
http://www.vh.org/welcome

This site includes information on treatments and management of the disease. It offers links to other Web sites on related topics. It also has pharmacological and other worksheets.

—— Alzheimer's Research Forum:
http://www.alzforum.org

This site has research information both for professionals in the health field and for patients.

—— Brain Food—Ginkgo Biloba:
http://www.china-guide.com/health/ginkgo.html

This site summarizes gingko's possible uses for Alzheimer's.

—— Herbal Remedies for Alzheimer's:
http://www.innerself.com/magazine/Herbs/Herbal_Remedies

This Web site is for those people who want to try something new. It offers herbal remedies and medicine to alleviate some symptoms of Alzheimer's. Visit this site to see if it is right for you.

—— Reishi and Ganoderma Lucidurn: Anti-inflammatory Agents for Alzheimer's:
http://www.Kyotan.com/lectures

William B. Stavinoha presents his investigation of the anti-inflammatory properties of Reishi and Ganoderma Lucidurn in the treatment of Alzheimer's. The site has research information on these products and links to related articles.

Financial Information and Products You Can Use

—— Alzheimer's, Day Care, Nursing Homes, and Medicaid:
http://www.rvralzheimers.com/page_4.htm

This Web site gives a brief summary of Medicaid. The purpose of the Web site is to invite you to seek help from the writer, Robert V.

Rowe. He wrote a book that gives a step-by-step account of how he got his wife into a nursing home and got Medicaid financial support.

— Alzheimer's Store:
http://thealzheimerstore.com
    This site lists products caregivers can use.

Resources (Books, Videotapes, and Other Resources)

— Alzheimer's Books:
http://members.aol.com/ctgabe/booksalz.htm
    This Web site contains the newest listings of Alzheimer's books. It even has a link to Amazon.com so you can order any book you are interested in.

— Resources on Alzheimer's Disease:
http://www.alzheimerbooks.com
    This Web page lists links to resources like the following: Elder Books sells books that are written in a user-friendly, nontechnical style. They provide key information and hands-on guidance to caregivers. The Alzheimer's Support Group Gray's Harbor (WA) is a Web site that has videotapes, resources, hotlines, and links to other Web sites.

INDEX

acetylcholine, 8, 146
activities, 38–39, 148; caregiver's, after patient death, 84; physical, 39, 84
agitation, 7, 17
agnosia, 5
aluminum, 4
Alzheimer's Association, 20, 21, 149
Alzheimer's disease: caregiver acceptance of, 3, 18; causes of, 3; diagnosis of, 1–12, 147; effects of, 13–23; environmental factors in, 3; genetic factors in, 3, 10–11; incidence of, 4; progressive nature of, 1–12; questions about, 137–150; research on, 7–8; stages of, 6–7; symptoms of, 3, 5; treatment for, 1–12
American Health Care Association, 150
amyloid protein, 3
anger, 54
annuities, 63, 68, 124
anti-inflammatory agents, 9, 11
antioxidants, 9
anxiety, 15
aphasia, 5
apraxis, 5
Aricept (donepezil HCl), 8, 146
aspirin, 8, 9

attorneys, elder law, 61–62, 71, 141
autopsy, 76

bathing, xii; aids for, 24, 25; assisting, 25; support rails, 24
behavior: changes in, 56; defensive, 6; medication and, 16, 17; repetitive, 7, 143, 145; "sundowning syndrome," 143; triggers for, 17; unacceptable, 17, 144; uncooperative, 27, 142; violent, 48
bereavement groups, 82–83
blood pressure, 17, 39, 126

caregiver(s): burnout in, 19; children as, 88–118; controlling sadness in, 40–41, 48; coping strategies for, 44; counseling for, 21–22, 148; delegation of responsibilities by, 44; eating habits of, 18; end-of-life choices for, 129; estate planning and, 122–125; financial planning for, 69–71; getting help for, 24–35, 137–138; management strategies for, 42–44; medication for, 17–18; after patient's death, 81–87, 120–132; personal time for, 19; privacy for, 144; support for, 19, 36–46; and time for self, 18

ABOUT THE AUTHOR

Rosette Teitel was born in France at the beginning of the Second World War. She and her mother came to the United States in 1946.

After she graduated college with honors in 1961 and earned a master's degree in French literature in 1963, she began her career by teaching French and Spanish in secondary school. She then became a teacher of English as a second language in 1976 after her French teaching position was eliminated during New York City's fiscal crisis. She learned that you can indeed make lemonade when life hands you lemons, and she found her work with immigrant teenagers even more rewarding than teaching French.

When her husband, Newton, was diagnosed with vascular dementia, she began to understand some of the puzzling behavior he had been exhibiting for a number of years. When he was not able to take care of himself anymore, she found herself frazzled and seeking help and advice wherever she could. It was in her Alzheimer's support group that she said, "There really should be a book out there to answer our questions."

When Newton died, she wrote this book. Her goal was to guide, support, and enlighten the caregivers of those who contracted Alzheimer's or other dementias. The teacher in her wanted to share the survival skills and practical advice she had acquired the hard way. It is her hope that *The Handholder's Handbook* will make life a little easier and inspire the reader to overcome adversity and believe in a brighter tomorrow.

She currently lives in Queens, New York, where she continues to teach on a volunteer basis and works as a mentor for new teachers. Besides participating in a circuit training fitness program, she is active in charitable organizations and often travels to the West Coast to visit her children.